THE PEGAN

DIET

COOKBOOK

{A Beginner's Guide}

Recipes to help you reverse disease optimize health, longevity, and performance.

By

Kim Cox

The Pegan Diet Cookbook
{A Beginner's Guide}

Disclaimer:

The information provided in this book is designed to provide helpful information on the subjects discussed. The publisher and author are not responsible for any specific health or allergy needs that may require medical supervision and are not liable for any damages or negative consequences from any treatment, action, application or preparation, to any person reading or following the information in this book.

Table of Contents

The Pegan Diet Cookbook
{A Beginner's Guide}

INTRODUCTION:

What is the pagan diet?

The pegan diet combines key principles from vegan and paleo diets based on the fact that nutrient-dense, whole foods can reduce inflammation, balance blood sugar, and enhance optimal health.

The pegan diet is unique and has its own set of guidelines. It's less restrictive than either a paleo or vegan diet by itself.

Main emphasis is placed on vegetables and fruit, but intake of small to moderate amounts of meat, nuts, certain fish, seeds, and some legumes is also permitted. Moreover, heavily processed oils, sugars, and grains are discouraged — but still acceptable in very small quantity.

However, the pegan diet is not designed as a typical, short-term diet. Instead, it targeted to be more sustainable so that you can follow it indefinitely.

Remember, the paleo and vegan diets both have been in the spotlight in recent years for their independent approaches to food and health. We probably think of them as polar opposites, with paleo focusing on meats our ancestors theoretically ate and veganism opting out of animal products altogether. A relatively new eating plan targeted to showing that meat-heavy paleo and veggie-centric veganism can coexist in a single diet.

In addition, the pegan diet emphasizes nutrient-rich fruits, vegetables, and healthy fats, it may help prevent disease, reduce inflammation and promote heart health.

The pegan diet (as in, paleo + vegan), was propounded by celebrity functional medicine doctor Mark Hyman, M.D., purports to offer the best of both worlds. Moreover, the diet advises filling 75 percent of your plate with plant-based foods and 25 percent with lean, sustainably raised meats. According to Dr. Hyman, eating this way can reduce the risk of chronic disease, curb inflammation, and promote general health.

Foods to eat and food to avoid

The pegan diet targeted strongly on whole foods, or foods that have undergone little to no processing before they make it to your plate.

However, the pegan diet is made up of 75 percent fruits and vegetables. The remaining 25 percent is divided basically among eggs, meats, and healthy fats, such as nuts and seeds. Some legumes and gluten-free whole grains may be permitted in limited quantities.

The bottom line of a pegan diet include choosing foods with a low glycemic load; vegetables, eating lots of fruits, nuts, and seeds (approximately three-quarters of your daily intake), choosing grass-fed or sustainably raised meats when you do eat meat; avoiding chemicals, pesticides, additives, and GMOs, Dairy, Gluten, Gluten-free grains, Legumes, Sugar, Refined oils. Most of these foods are forbidden due to their perceived impact on blood sugar and/or inflammation in your body. Plenty of healthy fats like omega-3s and unsaturated fat; and eating organically and locally.

The bottom line

First, the pegan diet is based mainly on paleo and vegan principles — though it encourages some meat consumption.

Moreover, it emphasizes whole foods, especially vegetables, while largely prohibiting gluten, most grains, dairy, and legumes.

It's rich in various nutrients that can enhance optimal health but may be too restrictive for many people.

Give this diet a try to see how your body responds. However, if you're already paleo or vegan and are interested in modifying your diet, I suggest the pegan diet may be easier to adjust to.

THE PEGAN RECIPES FOR A BETTER AND HEALTHIER YOU

BREAKFAST AND DESSERT RECIPES

CHOCOLATE COCONUT PALEO GRANOLA (GF + VEGAN)
INGREDIENTS

1 cup of pumpkin seeds (pepitas)

2 tablespoons of chia seeds

¼ cup of (about 60g) honey (or better still maple, to keep vegan)

2 teaspoons of vanilla extract

¼ cup of dark chocolate (chopped)

2 cups of raw almonds (or a mixture of your favorite nuts)

1 cup of (about 60g) flaked coconut, unsweetened

3 tablespoons (about 15g) cocoa powder

⅓ Cup of coconut oil (about 70g)

½ teaspoon of sea salt

Directions:

1. First, soak almonds and pepitas in water with a pinch of salt overnight or for about 8 hours.
2. After which you soaking the nuts first removes the enzyme inhibitors, making them easier to digest.

3. Meanwhile, heat the oven to 250°F.
4. After that, drain and rinse the nuts and dry them with a cloth towel.
5. Then you chop the nuts into small pieces and chunks, or place the nuts in the bowl of a food processor and pulse briefly until just coarsely chopped. {NOTE: I chopped them so that not all of the nuts were the same size for variety, but do whichever see fit!}
6. Furthermore, in large bowl, stir together the chopped nuts, chia seeds, flaked coconut, and cocoa powder.
7. At this point, add the melted coconut oil, honey, vanilla extract and sea salt and stir until all of the dry ingredients are completely coated in the wet ingredients.
8. Then place the granola on a Silpat or parchment-lined baking sheet and bake for about 2 ½ to 3 hours, stirring every ½ hour.
9. Finally, let cool slightly, and stir in the chopped dark chocolate
10. Then, let cool completely, and enjoy!
11. Make sure you store in the refrigerator.

NOTE: Try making your own Paleo Chocolate if you want to keep Paleo & refined sugar free.

Egg Breakfast Muffins

Ingredients

1 cup of diced broccoli

Salt and pepper {to taste}

8 eggs

1 cup of diced onion

1 cup of diced mushrooms

Directions

1. Meanwhile, heat oven to 350 degrees F.
2. After which you dice all vegetables. {NOTE: you can add more or less of any of them, but keep the overall portion of vegetables the same for best results}.
3. After that, in a large mixing bowl, whisk together eggs, salt, vegetables, and pepper.
4. Then pour mixture into a greased muffin pan, the mixture should evenly fill 8 muffin cups.
5. At this point, bake 18-20 minutes, or until a toothpick inserted in the middle comes out clean.
6. Finally, you serve and enjoy!

NOTE: Leftovers can be saved in the refrigerator throughout the week.

Easy and Delicious Sausage Frittata

Ingredients:

1 medium sweet potato {peeled and grated}

10 eggs

Pepper {to taste}

1 pound of mild Italian sausage (NOTE: I used our fresh pork in the freezer)

4 green onions {diced}

3 tablespoons of coconut oil

Directions:

1. First, in a large oven proof skillet, heat the coconut oil over medium heat.
2. After which you crumble in the sausage (remember to remove from casing if necessary) and brown.
3. After that, add the shredded sweet potato and cook until the potatoes are tender.
4. Then, add the diced green onion and sauté together with the sausage and sweet potatoes for another 2-3 minutes.
5. Furthermore, evenly spread the sausage mixture over the bottom of the pan.
6. At this point, whisk together the eggs, and pour evenly over the meat, sweet potato, and green onion mixture.
7. This is when you sprinkle all over with black pepper.
8. Then, cook for about 3 minutes or until bubbly and you can see that the edges of the frittata are almost done.
9. Finally, transfer to the oven and cook under the broiler on low until the frittata is cooked all the way through.
10. Enjoy!

SIMPLE BLUEBERRY MUFFINS

SERVES 8-10

Ingredients

1 cup of almond meal/almond flour

½ cup of raw honey

1/3 cup of coconut oil {melted}

½ teaspoon of baking powder

½ cup of fresh blueberries

1 cup of almond butter

3 eggs {whisked}

1/3 cup of unsweetened shredded coconut

½ teaspoon of baking soda

¼ teaspoon of sea salt

A pinch of cinnamon

Directions:

1. Meanwhile, heat your oven to 350 degrees.
2. After which you mix all ingredients together in a bowl. {NOTE: If you're good at baking, you'll know to mix the dry then the wet ingredients then mix together, but I do all the ingredients together and it works perfectly}.
3. After that, place ingredients into 8-10 silicone muffin cups in a muffin tin. Or better still you can use muffin tin paper liners.
4. Then, bake for 15-20 minutes. {Remember to keep an eye on it, they will puff up and look adorable}.
5. Enjoy.

PALEO ALMOND ZUCCHINI BREAD

TIPS:

This recipe is slightly crunchy on the outside and super moist on the inside and the perfect way to use up summer zucchini.

INGREDIENTS

1 ½ cups of almond flour (or better still a combination of almond and cashew flour)

1 ½ teaspoons of baking soda

½ teaspoon of salt

1 teaspoon of cinnamon

1 cup of grated zucchini, squeezed of excess water then measured to 1 cup

3 eggs

3 tablespoons of maple syrup

1 large banana {mashed}

1 tablespoon of melted coconut oil

DIRECTIONS:

1. Meanwhile, heat oven to 350 degrees and line a loaf pan with parchment paper.
2. After which you whisk together dry ingredients in a large bowl.
3. After that, add wet ingredients except zucchini and whisk until thoroughly combined.
4. Then, add zucchini and stir until combined.
5. At this point, pour batter into parchment lined loaf pan.

6.   Furthermore, bake for about 35 minutes until top is browned and center of the bread is set.

7.   After that, remove from oven and let cool in the pan on a wire rack for 5 minutes.

8.   Finally, remove bread from loaf pan by pulling on the sides of the parchment paper and place back on the wire rack to cool fully before slicing.

Paleo Strawberry Donuts (Nut/Grain/Dairy/Gluten Free)

SERVES: 1 dozen

CATEGORY: Dessert

PREP TIME: 30 mins

COOK TIME: 20 mins

INGREDIENTS:

3 tablespoons of coconut oil or ghee {melted}

¼ cup of honey

1 teaspoon of pure vanilla extract

¼ cup of freeze dried strawberries, ground to a powder

¼ teaspoon of sea salt

4 large eggs {room temperature}

½ cup of coconut milk, warm

1 teaspoon of apple cider vinegar

½ cup of coconut flour

½ teaspoon of baking soda

Topping

2 tablespoons of coconut butter

¼ cup of freeze dried strawberries {coarsely ground}

1 ounce raw cacao butter {melted}

1 teaspoon of honey

DIRECTION:

1. Meanwhile, heat a doughnut maker. Remember, if using a doughnut pan, preheat the oven to 350F and grease the pan liberally with butter.
2. After that, using a stand mixer or electric hand mixer, beat the eggs with the coconut oil on medium-high speed until creamy.
3. After which you add the vinegar, milk, honey, and vanilla and beat again until combined.
4. Furthermore, using a fine mesh sieve or sifter, sift the remaining dry ingredients into the bowl.
5. At this point, beat on high until smooth.
6. This is when you scoop the batter into a large Ziploc bag, seal the top, and snip one of the bottom corners.
7. Then, pipe the batter into the doughnut mold, filling it completely.
8. Finally, cook until the doughnut machine indicator light goes off.

NOTE: for the oven, bake for 17 minutes.

9. After which you remove the doughnuts and cool on a wire rack.
10. Feel free to trim if necessary.

Directions in making the glaze

1. First, mix the coconut butter, cacao butter, and honey in a shallow bowl.
2. After which you place in the freezer for 5 minutes to thicken.
3. Then, once the donuts are completely cooled, dip them in the glaze then dip the tops in the ground up strawberries.
4. Finally, place in the refrigerator for 20 minutes to allow the glaze to set.

Loco Moco

Ingredients:

2 precooked hamburger patties

2 cups of beef broth or better still stock

2 tablespoons of potato starch

2 scoops of white rice or better still cauliflower rice

4 eggs

1 teaspoon of black pepper

Directions:

1. First you make the brown gravy.
2. After which you bring the broth/stock to a light boil, adding the black pepper, and let it simmer while you create your thickener.
3. After that, in a small bowl add the potato starch and a little water, enough to make a milky-looking liquid.
4. At this point, you slowly pour it into the broth, stirring as it thickens.
5. Furthermore, once the gravy looks good, it's time to put it all together.
6. After that, fry up your eggs, leaving the yolks a little gooey.
7. Then, put one scoop of rice on a plate or in a bowl, add the hamburger, then the eggs, and cover it with a scoop or two of gravy.
8. Finally, repeat the process for the next loco moco, and you're good to go!

Pumpkin spice muffins with maple butter frosting

Prep time 15 mins

Cook time 30 mins

Serves: 8-10 muffins

Ingredients For the muffins

¾ cup of full-fat coconut milk or better still heavy cream

1 ½ teaspoons of vanilla extract

½ cup of coconut flour (preferably from Tropical Traditions)

1 teaspoon of pumpkin pie spice

4 eggs {lightly beaten}

¼ cup of canned pumpkin purée

½ cup of blanched almond flour (preferably from nuts.com)

½ teaspoon of baking soda

¼ teaspoon of sea salt (I prefer Redmond)

Ingredients for the maple butter frosting

1. ¼ cup of coconut butter, softened in the microwave or a bath of warm water on the stove (preferably from Tropical Traditions where it's known as coconut cream concentrate; NOTE: Artisanal and Nutiva are also good and can be found at the store)
2. 1 Tablespoon of maple syrup

Optional recipe: shaved chocolate to garnish (fancy)

Directions for the muffins

1. Meanwhile, heat oven to 350°
2. After which you combine the wet ingredients (coconut milk, eggs, pumpkin purée, and vanilla) in one bowl. Mix thoroughly.
3. After that you combine the dry ingredients (coconut flour, almond flour, baking soda, salt and spices) in another bowl. Mix thoroughly.
4. At this point, add the wet ingredients to the dry and mix until a wet dough forms.
5. This is when you drop the dough into muffin cups to approximately two-thirds full.
6. Then, place a ramekin half-filled with water in the oven before adding the muffins (NOTE: it will help keep them moist)
7. Finally, bake for 30 minutes and remove from oven.
8. This is when you allow them to cool before adding frosting.

Direction for the frosting

1. First, combine softened coconut butter and maple syrup.
2. Then, once muffins are cooled, top with frosting and shaved chocolate, if you want.
3. Finally, to shave chocolate, just take some of the chocolate you definitely stockpile in your freezer and run it across a cheese grater.

STRAWBERRY PALEO PANCAKE RECIPE

Ingredients

2 eggs

½ teaspoon of nutmeg

¼ teaspoon of baking powder

Coconut oil for frying

1 ½ cups of finely ground almond meal flour

½ teaspoon of cinnamon

½ cup of pureed strawberries

¼ cup of coconut or better still almond milk

Directions:

1. First, mix all the ingredients except the coconut oil for frying.
2. After which you add the coconut oil to a frying pan and heat till melted.
3. After that, use ¼ cup batter to make each pancake.
4. Then, fry until golden brown on each side.
5. Finally, top with more pureed strawberries or real Vermont maple syrup.

JUMBO CHICKPEA PANCAKE

Yield 1 large or 2 smaller

Prep time 10 minutes

Cook time 10 minutes

1. A HIGH PROTEIN, FILLING VEGAN BREAKFAST OR LUNCH!
2. You should feel free to change up the mix-ins and toppings based on what you have in your fridge.
3. Remember, to prevent it from sticking to the skillet, be sure to spray the skillet liberally with olive oil before pouring on the batter. Also, I will suggest you chopping the veggies finely so they cook faster.

INGREDIENTS

¼ cup of finely chopped red pepper

¼ teaspoon of garlic powder

1/8 teaspoon of freshly ground black pepper

½ cup + 2 tablespoons water

1 green onion, finely chopped (about ¼ cup)

½ cup of chickpea flour (AKA garbanzo flour or besan)

¼ teaspoon of fine grain sea salt

¼ teaspoon of baking powder

A pinch of red pepper flakes (it is optional)

For serving: avocado, hummus, salsa, cashew cream (optional)

DIRECTIONS

1. First, prepare the vegetables and set aside.

2. Meanwhile, heat a 10-inch skillet over medium heat.
3. After that, in a small bowl whisk together the garlic powder, salt, chickpea flour, baking powder, peppers, and optional red pepper flakes.
4. After which you add the water and whisk well until no clumps remain. {NOTE: I like to whisk it for a good 15 seconds to create lots of air bubbles in the batter}.
5. Then you stir in the chopped vegetables.
6. Furthermore, when the skillet is pre-heated (NOTE: a drop of water should sizzle on the pan), spray it liberally with olive oil or other non stick cooking spray.
7. At this point, pour on all of the batter (if making 1 large pancake) and quickly spread it out all over the pan.
8. This is when you cook for 5-6 minutes on one side (timing will depend on how hot your pan is), until you can easily slide a pancake flipper/spatula under the pancake and it's firm enough not to break when flipping.
9. Remember, flip pancake carefully and cook for another 5 minutes, until lightly golden.

NOTE: be sure to cook for enough time as this pancake takes longer to cook compared to regular pancakes.

10. Finally, serve on a large plate and top with your desired toppings.
11. Remember, leftovers can be wrapped up and placed in the fridge.
12. Feel free to reheat on a skillet until warmed throughout.

TIP:

Note: you can make this recipe into 2 smaller pancakes if desired.

Blueberry Oatmeal Waffles

INGREDIENTS

1 tablespoon of baking powder

¼ teaspoon of ground allspice

1/3 cup of unsweetened applesauce

3 tablespoons of pure maple syrup

1 ½ cups of frozen blueberries

1 cup of white whole wheat flour

½ teaspoon of salt

1 cup of quick cooking oats

1 ½ cups of unsweetened almond milk (or better still your fave non-dairy milk)

2 tablespoons of canola oil

1 teaspoon of pure vanilla extract

DIRECTIONS

1. First, baking powder, sift flour, salt and allspice into a mixing bowl.
2. After which you mix in the oats.
3. After that, make a well in the center and add maple syrup, applesauce, milk, oil and vanilla.
4. At this point, stir with just until combined.
5. Then you let batter rest for about 5 minutes or so, it will thicken a bit.
6. This is when you fold in the blueberries.

{**NOTE:** don't worry too much about the blueberries bleeding into the batter, it's no biggie}.

7. In addition, cook in waffle iron according to manufacturer directions. NOTE: in my 8 inch waffle iron, I use a heaping 1/2 cup of batter.
8. Finally, remember to spray or brush the iron with oil in between each waffle.

Chocolate Hazelnut Spread

Serves: 1 cup spread

Ingredients

    1-2 tablespoons of hazelnut or better still vegetable oil

    2 tablespoons of high-quality cocoa powder

    ¼ teaspoon of vanilla

    1½ cup of hazelnuts, skinned

    ¾ cup of powdered sugar

    2 tablespoons of soy powder

Directions:

1. First, toast hazelnuts in oven (or better still toaster oven) at 350° for ~20 minutes, tossing them frequently so as not to burn the nuts.
2. Then, while still hot, grind in a blender until nuts break down into nut butter, adding vanilla and a little oil during the blending process.
3. At this point, once coarse nut butter has been formed, add cocoa powder, powdered sugar, and soy powder, adding more oil as preferred.
4. Finally, blend until spread reaches desired consistency.

Notes

1. Remember, the longer you blend, the smoother and thinner the spread will become.

2. Make sure you grind for a shorter period of time or add more powdered sugar for a thicker spread.

Toast with Refried Beans and Avocado Recipe

YIELD: Serves 2

ACTIVE TIME: 5 minutes

Ingredients

1 cup of homemade or better still store-bought vegan refried beans

Coarse sea salt such as Maldon or better still fleur de sel

2 slices sandwich bread

1 avocado {thinly sliced}

A few slivers white onion

Directions

1. First, toast bread to desired level of doneness.
2. After which you top with refried beans and avocado (feel free to mash with a fork if desired).
3. Finally, add slivered onions, sprinkle with salt, and serve.

SOFT + CHEWY BAKED GRANOLA BARS

Yield 10-12 bars

Prep time 10 minutes

Cook time 25 minutes

TIP:

1. Chewy, soft, dense, seedy, doughy, hearty, protein-and-fiber-packed granola bars, sweetened naturally with dates!
2. You can try them spread with nut or seed butter for a fun treat or just enjoy them plain.

INGREDIENTS

1 cup of water

½ cup of chia seeds

¼ cup of raw pumpkin seeds

1 teaspoon of cinnamon

¼ teaspoon of fine grain sea salt

¾ cup of gluten-free rolled oats, ground into flour

¾ cup of packed pitted Medjool dates

¼ cup of raw sunflower seeds

¼ cup of dried cranberries {finely chopped}

1 teaspoon of pure vanilla extract

DIRECTIONS

1.   Meanwhile, heat oven to 325F and line a 9-inch square pan with two pieces of parchment paper, one going each way.
2.   After that, add rolled oats into a high-speed blender.
3.   After which you blend on highest speed until a fine flour forms.
4.   At this point, add oat flour into a large bowl.
5.   This is when you add water and pitted dates into blender.
6.   Furthermore, allow the dates to soak for 30 minutes if they are a bit firm or your blender has a hard time blending date's smooth.
7.   Then, once they are soft, blend the dates and water until super smooth.
8.   After which you add all of the ingredients into the bowl with the oat flour and stir well until combined.
9.   In addition, scoop the mixture into the pan and spread it out with a spatula as evenly as possible.

NOTE: you can use lightly wet hands to smooth it down if necessary.

10.   Finally, bake at 325F for about 23-25 minutes, or until firm to the touch.
11.   Then, let cool in the pan for 5 minutes and then lift it out and transfer it to a cooling rack for another 5-10 minutes.
12.   This is when you slice and enjoy!

Feel free to freeze leftovers to preserve freshness.

Peanut Butter Granola

Ingredients

2 tablespoons of Honey (preferable Maple Syrup or any alternative is fine)

1 cup of Oats

¼ teaspoon of Cinnamon

¼ teaspoon of Vanilla

2 tablespoons of Peanut Butter (I prefer Better n' Peanut Butter)

Directions

1. Meanwhile, heat oven to 325 degrees, than spray cookie sheet with non-stick cooking spray and set aside.
2. After which you combine peanut butter and honey in a bowl and microwave until peanut butter melts (approximately 20 seconds). Stir.
3. After that, stir cinnamon and vanilla into peanut butter and honey mixture.
4. At this point, add oats and stir until oats are completely covered in peanut butter mixture.
5. Then, spread out oat mixture onto prepared cookie sheet and bake for about 7 – 8 minutes until granola is slightly browned.
6. Furthermore, let cool until granola is crunchy.
7. Finally, keep in mind that this is not a superhero breakfast. As for me, this would be a dessert... a nice occasional treat!

15-Minute Breakfast Sandwich

TIPS:

This recipe can be whipped up in just 15 minutes! Super flavorful!

Prep: 5 mins

Cook: 10 mins

Servings: 1

Ingredients

> 2 Tablespoons of vegan sausage patty, any brand leafy greens, spinach, kale, – to taste – optional
>
> 1 teaspoon of hot sauce, optional
>
> ¼ avocados {optional}
>
> 1 English muffin
>
> 1 slice of vegan cheese
>
> 1 teaspoon of strawberry jam
>
> 1 teaspoon of extra virgin olive oil for coating the pan, optional

Directions:

1. First, pop your English muffin in the toaster.
2. After which you grab your patty and cheese. {**NOTE**: if using microwave, cook patty one minute}.
3. After that, add cheese, heat another thirty seconds. Remember, if using skillet, I suggest you add oil to pan.
4. Then, warm skillet over high heat.
5. Furthermore, cook patty for one minute, flip and add cheese.
6. At this point, cook until cheese is melted, then turn off heat.

7.   This is when you slice open the English muffin.
8.   After which you add jam to toasted English muffin.
9.   Additionally, add the patty and melted cheese.
10.   Finally, add optional greens and avocado. Serve!

Warm and Nutty Cinnamon Quinoa Recipe

TIPS:

1. For me I used a red quinoa, but feel free to use whatever kind you like, white/buff colored seems to be the most common.
2. You can substitute low-fat soy milk for low fat milk, dark honey may replace the agave nectar, blueberries may replace the blackberries, and walnuts may replace the pecans.

Ingredients:

1 cup of water

2 cups of fresh blackberries {organic preferred}

4 teaspoons of organic agave nectar {such as Madhava brand}

1 cup of organic 1% low fat milk

1 cup of organic quinoa, (note: rinse quinoa)

½ teaspoon of ground cinnamon

1/3 cup of chopped pecans {toasted}

Directions:

1. First, combine water, milk, and quinoa in a medium saucepan.
2. After which you bring to a boil over high heat.
3. After that, reduce heat to medium-low; cover and simmer for about 15 minutes or until most of the liquid is absorbed.
4. Then, turn off heat; let stand covered 5 minutes.

5. At this point, stir in blackberries and cinnamon; transfer to four bowls and top with pecans.

6. Make sure you drizzle 1 teaspoon agave nectar over each serving.

Serves 4.

Remember, at this point, while the quinoa cooks, roast the pecans in a 350F degree toaster oven for about 5 to 6 minutes or in a dry skillet over medium heat for about 3 minutes.

Canal House Lentils

ACTIVE TIME 45 MINUTES

TOTAL TIME 1 HOURS

TIPS:

This recipe when cooked with aromatics and rich tomato sauce, lentils are anything but bland.

Ingredients

8 SERVINGS

1 medium leek, white and pale-green parts only {finely chopped}

1 tablespoon of tomato paste

2 tablespoons of reduced-sodium soy sauce

Thinly sliced scallions (optional; for serving)

2 tablespoons of olive oil

1 clove garlic {thinly sliced}

1 cup of green lentils {preferably French}

Kosher salt and freshly ground black pepper

Directions:

1. First, heat oil in a medium saucepan over medium heat.
2. After which you add garlic, leek, and tomato paste and cook, stirring often, until fragrant and tomato paste begins to darken, about 4 minutes.
3. After that, add lentils and 2½ cups water.

4. Then, bring to a boil; reduce heat, cover, and simmer, stirring occasionally, until lentils are tender, 45–55 minutes.

5. Furthermore, remove from heat and let sit, covered, 10 minutes.

6. At this point, add soy sauce and season with salt and pepper.

7. This is when you serve lentils topped with scallions, if desired.

NOTE: remember lentils can be made 5 days ahead. Cover and chill.

Luscious Indian Cream of Wheat- A Delicious Breakfast Treat

Prep Time: 2 minutes

Cook Time: 5 minutes

TIPS:

This recipe is a simple and elegant filling hot breakfast, flavored with Indian spices and pistachio nuts. And it's so easy to put together.

2 servings

Ingredients:

2 cups of Coconut Milk

½ cup + 1 tablespoon of pistachios (finely chopped)

1 teaspoon of coconut oil {optional}

1/3 cup of whole grain of Cream of Wheat

1 tablespoon of rose water

½ teaspoon of cardamom (powder)

3 tablespoons of maple syrup, brown sugar or 3 packets of Stevia

Directions:

1. First, bring coconut milk to a boil in saucepan, watching it carefully to prevent it from boiling over.
2. After which you gradually add whole grain cream of wheat, ½ cup of pistachios, rosewater, cardamom and sugar stirring constantly with wire whisk until well blended.
3. Make sure you whisk without stopping so that no lumps form.

4. After that, reduce heat to Low; drizzle the coconut oil (if using) and simmer, uncovered for 3 minutes or until thickened, stirring frequently.

5. Then, you transfer to serving bowls, and garnish with remaining pistachios before serving.

Healthy Carrot Cake Muffins

This recipe is perfect for breakfast or a clean eating dessert! No grains or refined sugar needed but you'd never tell- Paleo, gluten free and easy to make!

Prep Time5 minutes

Cook Time20 minutes

Servings12 muffins

Ingredients

- ½ teaspoon of baking soda

- 1 teaspoon of cinnamon

- ¼ cup of maple syrup

- 4 tablespoons of coconut oil softened (feel free to use butter)

- ¼ cup of walnuts {optional}

- 1 cup of cream cheese frosting

- 2 cups of almond flour blanched almond flour or better still superfine almond flour

- ¼ teaspoon of salt

- 1 teaspoon of all spice

- 3 large eggs

- 1 cup of carrots shredded

Directions:

1. Meanwhile, heat the oven to 180C/350F.
2. After which you grease a 12-count muffin tin and fill with muffin tins and set aside.

3. After that, in a large mixing bowl, mix together your dry ingredients and mix well.
4. Then, add your wet ingredients, except for your carrots and walnuts, and mix until combined.
5. At this point, fold through your carrots and walnuts.
6. This is when; you distribute the batter amongst the 12 muffin tins.
7. Finally, bake for 20-22 minutes, or until a skewer comes out mostly clean.
8. In addition, remove from the oven and allow to cool in the pan completely, before frosting.

Notes

If you want keto muffins, I suggest you replace the maple syrup with keto maple syrup. Honey and agave can also be used to.

Healthy Sticky Cinnamon Roll Baked Oatmeal
TIPS:

A delicious, comforting chock full of nutrients and flavor and topped with a healthy glaze! Quick, easy, and delicious, this baked oatmeal recipe is perfect for a wholesome vegan and gluten free breakfast!

Prep Time5 minutes

Cook Time35 minutes

Servings8 servings

Ingredients

Dry ingredients

> 1 cup of quick oats gluten free, if needed
>
> 2 teaspoons of baking powder
>
> 1 teaspoon of allspice
>
> 1 cup of milk of choice
>
> 1/3 cup of almond butter can sub for any nut butter, coconut oil or butter
>
> 2 cups of rolled oats gluten free {if needed}
>
> ½ cup of granulated sweetener of choice
>
> 1 tablespoon of cinnamon
>
> 2 large eggs for vegan version, sub for 2 flax eggs
>
> 1 teaspoon of vanilla extract

Ingredients for the Cinnamon Roll Glaze

4 tablespoons of coconut butter melted

Ingredients For the protein packed Cinnamon Roll Glaze

2 tablespoons of milk of choice to thin out

2 teaspoons of Cinnamon

1-2 scoops cinnamon protein powder

Directions:

1. Meanwhile, heat the oven to 180C/350F and line an 8 x 8-inch pan with parchment paper. Set aside.
2. After which, in a large mixing bowl, combine all the dry ingredients and set aside.
3. After that, in a separate bowl combine the milk, eggs, vanilla extract and almond butter.
4. Then, whisk until combined, add the wet mixture to the dry and mix until fully combined.

NOTE: if the mixture is crumbly, I suggest you add a dash more milk until a thick batter is formed.

5. At this point, transfer the cinnamon roll baked oatmeal mixture to the lined baking dish.
6. Then, bake for 35-40 minutes, or until golden brown on top.
7. Finally, remove baked oatmeal and allow cooling for 5 minutes, before glazing, if desired.

Healthy Flourless Blueberry Breakfast Muffins

TIPS:

This recipe is fluffy on the inside and tender on the outside and the perfect, filling and energizing breakfast or snack option! Made with no oil, butter, flour or sugar, it an easy recipe which are completely vegan, refined sugar free, gluten free, dairy free and come with a tested paleo/grain free option!

Servings 9

Ingredients

Ingredients for the Gluten Free/Vegan/Flourless version

- ½ cup of granulated sweetener of choice {I used a monk fruit sweetener}

- A pinch of sea salt

- 1 flax egg can sub for 1 large egg if you not vegan

- 1/4-1/2 cup of blueberries

- 2 cups of gluten free rolled oats ground into flour

- 1 tablespoon of baking powder

- 1 cup of milk of choice

- 1 teaspoon of vanilla extract

- 6 Tablespoons of smooth cashew butter can sub for any nut butter of your choice

Ingredients for the Paleo option

- 1 cup of unsweetened applesauce

- ¼ cup of maple syrup can sub for honey or agave

Vanilla extract

1/4-1/2 cup of blueberries

½ cup of coconut flour

1/2 teaspoon of baking soda

¼ cup of melted coconut oil can sub for any nut butter of choice

4 large eggs whisked lightly

Directions:

1. Meanwhile, heat the oven to 350.
2. After which you grease a 10-12 count muffin tin generously with cooking spray/oil and set aside.
3. After that, in a large mixing bowl combine the dry ingredients and mix well.
4. Then, in a small bowl whisk the vanilla extract, milk, and egg/flax egg.
5. At this point, pour into the dry mixture.
6. Furthermore, add the melted nut butter (and maple syrup and applesauce for paleo option) and mix very well until a batter is formed.
7. Then, using a heaping ¼ cup, pour the muffin batter into the greased muffin tin.
8. After that, bake for around 30-35 minutes (NOTE: For paleo option, it can be up to 55 minutes, depending on the coconut flour) or until golden brown on top and a toothpick comes on clean.
9. Finally, remove from oven and allow cooling for 5 minutes in the muffin tin, before removing to a wire rack to cool completely.

Notes

Remember, muffins are freezer friendly and for optimum freshness, keep refrigerated.

Cinnamon Breakfast Cake

Tips:

This recipe tastes like a cinnamon bun and made in just one blender! No flour and no refined sugar, this cinnamon cake takes less than 30 minutes all up!

Prep Time5 minutes

Cook Time25 minutes

Servings9 Slices

Ingredients

Ingredients For the breakfast cake

- ½ cup of granulated sweetener of choice
- 1 tablespoon of cinnamon
- 1 cup of milk of choice {I prefer unsweetened almond milk}
- 6 tablespoons of almond butter
- 2 cups of rolled oats gluten free, if needed
- 1 tablespoon of baking powder
- 1/8 teaspoon of salt
- 1 teaspoon of vanilla extract
- 1 flax egg can use 1 large egg

Ingredients For the frosting

- 1 cup of cream cheese frosting

Directions:

1. Meanwhile, heat the oven to 180C/350F.
2. After which you grease an 8-inch cake pan with cooking spray and set aside.
3. Then, in a high speed blender or food processor, add your oats and blend until a powder like consistency remains.
4. After that, add the rest of your ingredients and blend until a thick batter remains.
5. At this point, transfer the batter to the greased cake pan.
6. Furthermore, bake for 25-30 minutes or until a skewer comes on clean.
7. Finally, remove from oven and allow to cool completely before frosting, if desired.

Notes

If you want to make a flax egg, I suggest you combine 1 tablespoon of ground flaxseed with 3 tablespoons water. Then, let sit for 10 minutes, for a gel to form.

Oatmeal Brownies

TIPS:

This recipe is thick, fudgy, and perfect for breakfast! Made with oat flour and naturally sweetened, they are packed with protein, fiber, and full of chocolate flavor!

Prep Time10 minutes

Cook Time30 minutes

Servings12 Brownies

Ingredients

> 1 ½ cups of cocoa powder
>
> ½ cup of peanut butter smooth and creamy
>
> 2/3 cup of maple syrup
>
> 1-2 cups of chocolate chopped, optional
>
> ½ cup + 2 tablespoons of oat flour
>
> ¼ teaspoon of salt
>
> 3/4 cup of coconut oil melted
>
> 1 cup of granulated sweetener of choice brown, coconut, or sugar free subs
>
> 4 large eggs can use vegan subs like flax eggs

Directions:

1.   Meanwhile, heat the oven to 180C/350F.
2.   After which you line an 8 x 8-inch pan with parchment paper and set aside.

3. After that, in a small bowl add your cocoa powder, oat flour, and salt, and mix well. Set aside.

4. Furthermore, in a separate bowl, whisk together your maple syrup, peanut butter, coconut oil, and granulated sweetener of choice.

5. Then, whisk together until combined and glossy.

6. At this point, add your eggs and whisk well.

7. This is when you combine your wet and dry ingredients and mix together until just combined.

8. In addition, fold through your chocolate, if using them.

9. After which you transfer the brownie batter into the lined pan.

10. Finally, bake the brownies for about 30-35 minutes, or until a skewer comes out clean from the center.

11. Then, let cool in the pan completely, before slicing.

Healthy Sweet Potato Breakfast Brownies

Thick, chewy and super fudgy brownies made with just five healthy ingredients and designed specifically for breakfast! These healthy sweet potato breakfast brownies are completely paleo, vegan, gluten free, and sugar free and packed with protein!

Prep Time5 minutes

Total Time20 minutes

Servings8 servings

Equipment

> **Keto Maple Syrup**
>
> **Sugar Free Chocolate Chips**
>
> **Mixing bowl**
>
> **Almond Butter**
>
> **Paleo Vegan Chocolate Chips**

Ingredients

> 1 cup of almond butter can substitute for any nut or seed butter of choice
>
> ½ cup of cocoa powder
>
> 1 serving healthy frosting of choice
>
> 2 cups of sweet potatoes pureed
>
> ¼ cup of sugar free maple syrup can sub for pure maple syrup
>
> ½ cup of chocolate chips of choice optional

Directions:

1. Meanwhile, heat the oven the 350 degrees Fahrenheit and lightly grease a small loaf pan (thicker brownies) or 8 x 8 inch pan (perfect for thicker frosting) and set aside.
2. After which, in a large mixing bowl combine all your ingredients and mix until fully incorporated.
3. After that, pour into the greased pan and bake for 20-22 minutes, or until a skewer just comes out clean.
4. Then, remove from oven and allow cooling in the pan completely.
5. Furthermore, while brownies are cooling, prep your frosting of choice- See above the recipe card for the options (protein packed, coconut cream ganache, a chocolate bar of choice or homemade Nutella).

Remember, once brownies are cooled, frost and cut into pieces.

Notes

1. Make sure sweet potatoes are completely pureed; otherwise your brownies will have clumps.
2. These brownies contain no eggs, I suggest you remove them from the oven earlier than before they are done- They will be ultra fudgy this way.
3. Remember, brownies need to be kept refrigerated and are freezer friendly.

4 Ingredient No Bake Raw Flourless Brownies (Paleo, Vegan, Gluten Free)

TIPS:

These super rich recipes require no baking, use just 4 ingredients and are designed specifically for breakfast! They are completely naturally sweetened, protein-packed and are vegan, paleo, gluten free, dairy free and refined sugar free!

Prep Time2 minutes

Servings20 servings

Equipment

> **High speed blender**
>
> **Food Processor**
>
> **Mixing bowl**

Ingredients

> 2 cups of Medjool dates packed
>
> 1/4 teaspoon of sea salt Optional, but brings out the sweetness
>
> 4 cups of raw unsalted cashews {divided}
>
> ½ cup of cocoa powder
>
> 1-4 scoops of protein powder Optional

Ingredients for the Frosting:

> 1 serving classic frosting

1 serving protein frosting

Directions:

1. First, line an 8 x 6 loaf pan with parchment paper and set aside.
2. Then, in a high-speed blender (one which can pulse nuts) or food processor, add all your ingredients, except for half the nuts and process until almost completely smooth.
3. After that, add the rest of the nuts and blend until the nuts are roughly blended in.

NOTE: if you include protein powder, you may need some liquid to form batter.

4. Furthermore, transfer the thick brownie batter into the loaf pan and press firmly in place.
5. After which you place in the refrigerator while preparing the frosting of choice.
6. Finally, top no bake brownies with frosting of choice, top with a dash of sea salt and refrigerate for about 10-15 minutes, before slicing into even sized bars.

Notes

Remember, no Bake Breakfast Brownies are best kept refrigerated but are freezer friendly. For a super fudgy brownie, I suggest you enjoy at room temperature.

No Bake Vanilla Cake Batter Breakfast Cookies

TIPS:

However, one bowl and ten minutes is all you'll need to have dessert for breakfast- With a healthy makeover! This recipe is single serving, gluten, sugar and dairy free with a vegan option too!

Servings1

Ingredients

¼ cup of gluten free oat flour gluten free rolled oats ground to a flour

1-2 Tablespoons of sweetener of choice**

A pinch sea salt

¼ cup of gluten free oat bran

1 scoop of vanilla flavored protein powder*

2 Tablespoons of mild tasting nut butter of choice I used cashew butter and coconut butter

¼ teaspoons of vanilla essence/extract

1/4-1/2 cup of dairy free milk of choice {I prefer unsweetened vanilla almond milk}

Sprinkles optional

Directions:

1. First, line a large plate with baking paper and set aside.
2. After which in a large mixing bowl, combine the oat bran, protein powder, oat flour, sea salt and mix well. A

3. After that, add the nut butter of choice and mix through until the batter is very crumbly.
4. At this point, add the vanilla extract/essence and using a tablespoon, add the milk of choice until a very thick batter is formed. S
5. Then, stir through sprinkles and form into three to four large balls and place on the lined plate.
6. Furthermore, press firmly into a cookie shape and top with extra sprinkles.
7. Finally, eat immediately or for a firmer cookie (and ones which can be portable and left at room temperature), refrigerate or freeze for at least 30 minutes.

Notes

Remember, if you use an unflavored protein powder, up the vanilla essence to 1/2 teaspoon and ensure you add the sweetener of choice and secondly, if you're protein powder isn't overly sweet or you want a very sweet cookie, I suggest you add the sweetener of choice. It all depends on the protein powder you prefer, you may need more or less liquid.

No Bake Cookies and Cream Breakfast Bars

Prep Time5 minutes

Cook Time5 minutes

Total Time10 minutes

Servings12 servings

Ingredients

Ingredients For the cookies and cream bars

> ½ cup of coconut flour

> ½ cup of sunflower seed butter can sub for any nut or seed butter of choice

> ½ cup of unsweetened applesauce

> 1 cup of cookie pieces

> 2 cups of almond flour can sub for oat flour or better still another flour of choice

> ½ cup of vanilla protein powder {its optional}

> ½ cup of sticky sweetener of choice

> ¼ cup of liquid of choice *

Ingredients For the frosting

> 1 serving Frosting of your choice

Directions:

1. First, line a large 8 x 8 inch baking dish or loaf pan with tin foil or parchment paper and set aside.
2. After which in a large mixing bowl, add your dry ingredients and mix well. A
3. After that, add your wet ingredients, except for the cookie crumbles and liquid of choice.
4. Then, mix very well until a crumbly texture remains.
5. Furthermore, using a tablespoon, add milk of choice until a thick batter remains.
6. At this point, add chopped cookie pieces and mix well. A
7. This is when you add additional milk if necessary and transfer to the lined baking dish.
8. In addition, press firmly into place and refrigerate.
9. Finally, if using frosting, prep it now and spread over the breakfast bars.
10. Make sure you refrigerate until firm and slice into bars.

Notes

It depends on the protein powder and coconut flour, you'll likely need more. Make sure you adjust accordingly.

Cinnamon Roll Oatmeal

TIPS:

This recipe is delicious, healthy and hearty and tastes exactly like a cinnamon roll! However, this quick and easy cinnamon roll oatmeal recipe tastes like dessert and can be enjoyed hot or cold!

Prep Time2 minutes

Cook Time5 minutes

Servings1 serving

Ingredients

Ingredients For the oatmeal

> ¼ teaspoon of salt
>
> ½ tablespoon of Cinnamon
>
> 1-2 tablespoon of cream cheese dairy free {if needed}
>
> ½ cup of rolled oats gluten free {if needed}
>
> 2 tablespoons of granulated sweetener of choice
>
> 1 cup of milk of choice {I prefer unsweetened almond milk}

Directions:

1. First, in a saucepan or microwave safe bowl, combine the rolled oats, cinnamon, salt, sweetener of choice and milk of choice and simmer on medium until most of the liquid is absorbed. Remember, if adding protein powder, I suggest you add it here now.
2. After which you remove from heat and pour into a bowl.
3. Then, stir through the cream cheese and top with extra cinnamon

Notes

1.   If your oatmeal is too thick, I suggest you add extra milk to desired consistency.

2.   Remember, this can be batch made the night before and eaten hot/cold and can also be frozen- Simply thaw out and reheat.

3.   For even more protein, I suggest you add an extra scoop of protein powder but add extra dairy free milk to compensate.

4.   Feel free to use any sweetener of choice- erythritol, coconut sugar, white sugar, etc.

Healthy Vanilla Cake Batter Oatmeal

TIPS:

This recipe is smooth, creamy and delicious oatmeal which has the taste and texture of actual vanilla cake batter! This recipe can be enjoyed hot or cold and is suitable for those following a vegan, dairy free, gluten-free, and sugar free lifestyle!

Servings1

Ingredients

> A pinch of sea salt
>
> ½ teaspoon of vanilla extract
>
> 1 scoop of vanilla protein powder {optional but highly recommended}
>
> 1 Tablespoon of granulated sweetener of choice optional
>
> ½ cup of rolled oats I used gluten free rolled oats
>
> 1 Tablespoon of coconut flour sifted
>
> 1 large egg for a vegan option, sub for 1 flax egg- 1 Tablespoon flax + 3 Tablespoon water
>
> 1 ¼ cups of dairy free milk of choice divided
>
> Sprinkles to top {optional}

Directions:

1. First, combine oats, salt and 1 cup of milk in a saucepan or microwave safe bowl until most of the liquid is absorbed.
2. After which you whisk in the whole egg very well (or flax egg) and continue cooking for another 1-2 minutes, until oats are extremely fluffy.

3. After that, stir in the vanilla protein powder, sweetener of choice, vanilla extract and coconut flour until fully combined {NOTE: Oatmeal mixture should be extremely thick}.
4. Then, add in the extra ¼ cup of milk and ensure it is well mixed.
5. Furthermore, once this is done, refrigerate uncovered.
6. The next morning, I suggest you stir the oatmeal very well and top with nut butter/sprinkles etc. Reheat if desired.

Notes

1. However, if protein powder is sweetened, omit. The protein powder is optional- If you omit, I suggest you decrease the dairy free milk by ¼ cup.
2. Remember, if you don't have coconut flour; add a tablespoon of flax meal, oat flour or better still almond flour.

Healthy High Protein Snickers Overnight Oats

TIP:

This healthy recipe has all the best bits of a snickers candy/chocolate bar, minus the added fats, butter and nastiest AND packed with lots of protein! Because of the ingredients used, it is also completely vegan, gluten free, dairy free and sugar free!

Servings1

Ingredients

> 1 Tablespoon of coconut flour can sub for 1 Tablespoon oat flour or almond flour
>
> 1 scoop of vanilla protein powder {optional}
>
> A pinch sea salt
>
> 2 Tablespoons of crushed salted peanuts divided
>
> 1 Tablespoon of caramel sauce of choice sees above
>
> Sea salt {to garnish}
>
> ½ cup of gluten free rolled oats
>
> 1-2 Tablespoons of granulated sweetener of choice*
>
> 1 Tablespoon of ground flax can sub for chia seeds
>
> Drop vanilla extract
>
> 1/2-3/4 cup + milk of choice {I used unsweetened almond}
>
> 1 Tablespoon of chocolate sauce

Directions:

1. First, in a cereal bowl or small container, combine your rolled oats, vanilla protein powder, coconut flour, ground flax, sea salt and mix well. A

2. After which you add ½ cup first, vanilla extract and mix well. Remember, if mixture is too crumbly (it may be due to coconut flour and protein powder), I suggest you add extra dairy free milk until an inch or so remains above the oats.

3. At that, you add 1 tablespoon of the salted peanuts and refrigerate for at least an hour, or overnight.

4. Then, the next morning, remove- Oat mixture should be thick and creamy. If too thick, I suggest you add milk to thin out to desired consistency.

5. Finally, top with chocolate sauce, caramel sauce, extra tablespoon of salted peanuts and a dash of sea salt and enjoy!

Vegan Gluten Free Almond Joy Overnight Oatmeal

Tips:

This recipe has all the best bits of an almond joy candy bar in oatmeal form-Chocolate chips, almonds, and shredded coconut and it's protein packed and with a keto and low carb option!

Prep Time5 minutes

Cook Time5 minutes

Total Time10 minutes

Servings1 serving

Ingredients

- 1 tablespoon of coconut flour

- 1-2 tablespoons of granulated sweetener of choice

- 1/2-3/4 cup of coconut milk can use any milk of choice

- 1 tablespoon of chocolate chips of choice

- ½ cup of gluten free rolled oats

- 1 tablespoon of ground flaxseed

- 1 scoop vanilla protein powder {optional}

- 1 tablespoon of shredded unsweetened coconut

- 1/2 tablespoon of almonds

Keto Option

- 1 tablespoon of shredded unsweetened coconut

1 tablespoon of keto chocolate chips

1 serving keto oatmeal base

1/2 tablespoon of almonds

Directions:

1. First, in a cereal bowl or small container, combine your rolled oats, vanilla protein powder, ground flax, coconut flour, sea salt and mix well.
2. After which you add your milk of choice and mix well.
3. After that, slowly stir in half your coconut, chocolate chips and almonds and mix well.
4. Then, add extra milk if needed, and refrigerate.
5. However, the next morning or several hours later, I suggest you remove from the fridge.
6. Finally, add extra milk before topping with the rest of the coconut, almonds and chocolate chips.

Keto/Paleo directions

1. First, prepare keto oatmeal base as directed.
2. Then, the next morning, stir in your almonds, coconut, and chocolate and mix well.
3. Finally, add extra milk if needed, and enjoy.

Healthy High Protein Golden Milk Overnight Oats

Tips:

This healthy recipe is creamy, comforting and full of flavor! It made with warming spices with healing properties; this recipe is naturally vegan, gluten free, dairy free and can be made sugar free!

Servings1

Ingredients

1 Tablespoon of coconut flour can sub for 1 Tablespoon of oat flour or almond flour

1 scoop of vanilla protein powder optional

A pinch sea salt

A pinch ginger

A drop vanilla extract

1- 2 Tablespoons of honey or maple syrup use a sugar free maple syrup to keep it sugar free

½ cup of gluten free rolled oats

1-2 Tablespoon of granulated sweetener of choice*

1 Tablespoon of ground flax can sub for chia seeds

A pinch black pepper OR cayenne pepper

Pinch turmeric

1/2-3/4 cup + unsweetened coconut milk, feel free to use any milk of choice

Directions:

1. First, in a cereal bowl or small container, combine your rolled oats, vanilla protein powder, coconut flour, sea salt, ground flax, pepper and ginger and mix well. A

2. After which you add ½ cup coconut milk first, vanilla extract and mix well. Remember, if mixture is too crumbly (it may be due to coconut flour and protein powder), I suggest you add extra coconut milk until an inch or so remains above the oats and refrigerate for at least an hour, or overnight.

3. Then, the next morning, remove oat mixture from the fridge- The oat mixture should be thick and creamy. Remember, if too thick; add more coconut milk to thin out to desired consistency.

4. Finally, stir through turmeric and swirl through the honey/maple syrup on top and enjoy!

Keto Chia Pudding (Vegan)

Tips:

1. This recipe is smooth, creamy, and perfect for a low carb breakfast!
2. 5 minutes prep and easy to customize in many ways- whole30, Vegan, and gluten free.

Prep Time5 minutes

Cook Time1 hour

Servings1 serving

Ingredients

Ingredients For the chia seed pudding

1 teaspoon of cinnamon

1 tablespoon of granulated sweetener of choice

3 tablespoons of chia seeds

1 cup of milk of choice {I prefer coconut milk}

Ingredients For the cinnamon roll coconut butter glaze

½ teaspoon of cinnamon

1 tablespoon of milk of choice

1 tablespoon of coconut butter melted

1 tablespoon of granulated sweetener of choice

Directions:

To make the chia seed pudding

1. First, in a small cereal bowl or glass, mix together your chia seeds, cinnamon, and milk of choice.
2. After which you refrigerate for at least an hour, or overnight to form a pudding.
3. Then, once thick, remove from fridge and top with toppings of choice

Directions on how to make glaze

First, combine all ingredients and mix through and drizzle on top.

Notes

1. Remember, if chia seed pudding is too thick, I suggest you add extra milk of choice when ready to eat.
2. Any keto sweetener of your choice can be used.
3. Make sure you store chia pudding in the refrigerator at all times.

Healthy Brownie Batter Chia Seed Pudding

Tips:

This thick, creamy and satisfying recipe is the perfect snack, dessert or breakfast! Made with wholesome ingredients and with barely any prep, it's naturally gluten free, vegan, dairy free, paleo, sugar free and packs a protein punch!

Servings1

Ingredients

Ingredients For the pudding

> 1 Tablespoon of cocoa powder raw cacao for whole30 option
>
> 1 cup of milk of choice {I prefer unsweetened almond milk}
>
> 2 Tablespoons of chocolate sauce of choice divided (see notes above for sugar free and paleo options) - For whole30, I suggest you sprinkle with raw cacao powder, coconut shreds and cinnamon.
>
> 3 Tablespoons of white or black chia seeds
>
> 1 Tablespoon of protein powder of choice optional
>
> 1 Tablespoon of granulated sweetener of choice OR liquid sweetener of choice omit for whole30 option
>
> 2 Tablespoons of chocolate chips of choice divided (sugar free, dairy free or standard) - Omit for whole30 option

Optional protein packed chocolate glaze

> 1 Tablespoon of granulated sweetener of choice
>
> Milk to thin out
>
> 2 Tablespoons of chocolate protein powder

1 teaspoon of cocoa powder

Directions:

Directions to make the chia seed pudding

1. First, in a small cereal bowl or glass, mix together your chia seeds, cocoa powder, protein powder and add in your milk of choice and sweetener of choice and mix very well until a liquid mixture remains. S
2. After that, stir through one tablespoon of the chocolate chips and chocolate sauce and refrigerate for at least an hour, or overnight to form a pudding.
3. Then, once thick, remove from fridge and top with optional glaze, chocolate sauce and chocolate chips.

Directions to make glaze

All you do is mix all ingredients and add milk until a glaze is formed.

Notes

Remember, if chia pudding is too thick, I suggest you add a dash more milk of choice the next morning.

Delectable Lunch Recipes

Sweet Potato Noodles with Brussels sprouts and Lentil Ragu

15 MINPREP TIME

25 MINCOOK TIME

Ingredients:

> 1 bay leaf
>
> 3 medium sweet potatoes {peeled, Blade D, noodles trimmed}
>
> ¼ teaspoon of garlic powder
>
> 1 small red onion {peeled and diced}
>
> 2 celery stalks {diced}
>
> 2.5 cups of shredded Brussels sprouts
>
> Grated parmesan cheese, if desired (to garnish)
>
> ½ cup of dry brown lentils
>
> 1.5 cups of water
>
> 2 tablespoons of extra virgin olive oil
>
> Salt and pepper
>
> 2 garlic cloves {minced}
>
> 2 small carrots {diced}
>
> 1.5 cups of Victoria Fine Foods Organic Marinara sauce (or similar jarred sauce)

Chopped parsley to garnish

Directions:

1. First, place the lentils, bay leaf, and water in a small saucepan over high heat and bring to a boil.
2. Then, once boiling, reduce heat to low, cover and let simmer for 15 minutes or until lentils are cooked through, adding more water as needed.
3. In the meantime, cook the sweet potato noodles.
4. After which you heat half of the olive oil in a large skillet over medium-high heat.
5. At this point, once oil is shimmering, add the sweet potato noodles and season with salt, garlic powder, and pepper.
6. This is when you cook, tossing occasionally, until cooked through and al dente, about 7 minutes.
7. Furthermore, when done, transfer noodles to a plate and tent with foil to keep warm.
8. After that, place the skillet back over medium-high heat and add the remaining olive oil.
9. Then, once oil is shimmering, add the onions, celery, garlic, and carrots and cook for 5 minutes until vegetables soften.
10. After which you add the Brussels sprouts and cook until browned, about 5 minutes.
11. In addition, add the lentils and tomato sauce and let cook for 5 more minutes, letting flavors mend together.
12. Finally, divide the sweet potato noodles into bowls and top with equal amounts of the ragu.
13. Make sure you garnish with parsley and cheese (if desired.)

Satay Style Spiral zed Vegetables Stir Fry {Paleo, Vegan}

DESCRIPTION

INGREDIENTS

1 cup of chopped Napa cabbage (feel free to use more if you want more veggies)

1 tablespoon of sesame oil

½ to 1 teaspoon of red chili flakes

1 teaspoon of agave nectar (it is optional)

¼ teaspoon of five spices Asian seasoning

Black pepper {to taste}

3 zucchini and/or yellow squash (**NOTE:** spiral zed into noodles)

¼ cup of chopped red or green onion

3 to 4 tablespoons of creamy nut or seed butter (**NOTE:** Cashew butter or almond butter. Make sure you adjust according to how much zucchini you use).

2 tablespoons of tamari or gluten free soy sauce

1 teaspoon garlic (minced)

Dash of sea salt

Optional topping – Asian chili sauce (gluten free)

Directions:

1. First, spiralize your zucchini and squash.
2. After which you clean and press excess water from zucchini with paper towel.

3. After that, chop your cabbage and red onion, and then set aside.
4. At this point, heat a wok or skillet to medium high or high and add in your creamy nut butter. (NOTE: Make sure it's smooth or slightly creamy beforehand), sesame oil, garlic, tamari, and chili flakes.
5. Furthermore, mix all together and let is melt in pan on medium to medium low, until combined.
6. Then, toss in your onion and cabbage and stir fry on medium high for 1-2 minutes.
7. In addition, add in your zucchini noodles and remaining seasoning and spices.
8. After that, stir fry all together for a few minutes until veggies are cooked and coated but not soggy.
9. This is when you remove and garnish with more chili flakes, green onion, cilantro, Thai pepper, and splash of lime juice if desired.
10. Finally, drizzle with optional Asian chili sauce for a nice kick!
11. Remember, this recipe is great with cooked chicken or beef or shrimp! Or by itself!
12. Make sure you keep well in fridge in airtight container for up to 3-4 days.

NOTES

For whole 30 option, I suggest you omit agave or honey, and use coconut aminos in place of gluten-free soy sauce.

Directions on how to stir fry spiral zed veggies without them becoming too watery or soggy

1. First, bake the zoodles. Or better still let them sit in a colander with a pinch of sea salt. {**NOTE:** this will extract a lot of the water and then you can press them dry}.
2. However, if baking, preheat the oven to 350 degrees F.
3. After that, arrange the veggies noodles on a very large baking sheet or casserole dish.
4. Then, space them out so they are not clumped. T
5. At this point, toss with a bit of kosher salt.
6. Finally, bake for 10-15 minutes and then place on a towel and press dry.

ROT CROWD-PLEASING VEGAN CAESAR SALAD

Yield 6 small bowls

Prep time 45 minutes

Cook time 35 minutes

Tips:

1. This recipe is a delicious, creamy vegan Caesar salad and everyone who's tried it goes absolutely nuts over it, and it's my most popular salad recipe.
2. However, to take it over the top, I suggest you garnish the salad with a generous amount of crunchy Roasted Chickpea Croutons and a delectable Nut and Seed Parmesan Cheese for the ultimate vegan Caesar salad.

INGREDIENTS

INGREDIENTS FOR THE ROASTED CHICKPEA CROUTONS:

1 teaspoon (about 5 mL) extra-virgin olive oil

1/8 to ¼ teaspoon of cayenne pepper (it is optional)

1 (about 14-ounce/398 mL) can chickpeas (or 1 ½ cups cooked), drained and rinsed

½ teaspoon of fine grain sea salt

½ teaspoon of garlic powder

INGREDIENTS FOR THE CAESAR DRESSING (MAKES 3/4-1 CUP):

¼ cup (about 60 mL) water

1 tablespoon (about 15 mL) lemon juice

½ teaspoon of garlic powder

½ tablespoon (about 7.5 mL) vegan Worcestershire sauce (I prefer Wizard's gluten-free brand)

½ teaspoon of fine grain sea salt and pepper, or to taste

½ cup of raw cashews {soaked overnight}

2 tablespoons (about 30 mL) extra-virgin olive oil

½ tablespoon (about 7.5 mL) Dijon mustard

1 small garlic clove (feel free to add another if you like it super potent)

2 teaspoons of capers

INGREDIENTS FOR THE NUT AND SEED PARMESAN CHEESE:

2 tablespoons of hulled hemp seeds

1 tablespoon of nutritional yeast

Fine grain sea salt {to taste}

1/3 cup of raw cashews

1 small garlic clove

1 tablespoon (about 15 mL) extra-virgin olive oil

½ teaspoon of garlic powder

INGREDIENTS FOR THE LETTUCE:

2 small heads romaine lettuce (about 10 cups chopped)

1 small/medium bunch lacinato kale, destemmed (about 5 cups chopped)

DIRECTIONS

1. First, soak cashews in a bowl of water overnight, or for at least a few hours.
2. After which you drain and rinse.
3. After that, roast chickpea croutons: meanwhile, heat oven to 400°F (200°C).
4. After which you drain and rinse chickpeas.
5. After that, place chickpeas in a tea towel and rub dry (NOTE: it's okay if some skins fall off).
6. Then, place onto large rimmed baking sheet.
7. Furthermore, drizzle on oil and roll around to coat.
8. This is when you sprinkle on the garlic powder, salt, and optional cayenne; toss to coat.
9. In addition, roast for 20 minutes at 400°F (200°C), then gently roll the chickpeas around in the baking sheet.
10. Finally, roast for another 10 to 20 minutes, until lightly golden. {NOTE: They will firm up as they cool}.

Directions on how to prepare the dressing:

1. First, add the cashews and all other dressing ingredients (except salt) into a high-speed blender, and blend on high until the dressing is super smooth. Remember, you can add a splash of water if necessary to get it blending.
2. After which you add salt to taste and adjust other seasonings, if desired; set aside.

Directions on how to prepare the Parmesan cheese:

1. First, add cashews and garlic into a mini food processor and process until finely chopped.
2. After that, add in the rest of the ingredients and pulse until the mixture is combined; salt to taste.

Directions on how to prepare the lettuce:

1. First, destem the kale and then finely chop the leaves.
2. After which you wash and dry in a salad spinner.
3. After that, place into extra-large bowl.
4. Then, chop up the romaine into bite-sized pieces.
5. At this point, rinse and then spin dry.
6. Furthermore, place into bowl along with kale. {NOTE: you should have roughly 5 cups chopped kale and 10 cups chopped romaine}.

How to Assemble:

1. First, add dressing onto lettuce and toss until fully coated.
2. After which you season with a pinch of salt and mix again.
3. Finally, sprinkle on the roasted chickpeas and the Parmesan cheese.
4. Make sure you serve immediately.

TIP:

Remember, the dressing thickens when chilled, so be sure to leave it at room temperature to soften before using.

Sesame Sweet Potato Noodles

Prep Time 5 minutes

Cook Time 15 minutes

Servings 2

Ingredients

1 tablespoon of olive oil

1 tablespoon of toasted sesame oil

2 teaspoons of raw honey or maple syrup

¼ teaspoon of salt

1 tablespoon of sesame seeds

1 large sweet potato

2 tablespoons of tahini paste

2 tablespoons of raw apple cider vinegar

A pinch crushed red pepper flakes

1 green onion {diced}

Directions:

1. First, cook the sweet potato in a 425-degree oven for 10 minutes (remember it will not be fully cooked at this point).
2. Then, while the potato cools enough to handle make the dressing.
3. After which, in a small bowl whisk together the vinegar, sesame oil, honey, red pepper flakes, tahini, and salt.
4. At this point, set the dressing aside.
5. Furthermore, spiralizer the sweet potato into noodles.

6. After that, in a medium sauté pan heat the olive oil and cook the sweet potato noodles for about 5 minutes (**NOTE:** I like them slightly crunchy but cook longer if desired).

7. Finally, toss in the dressing, green onions, and sesame seeds.

8. Make sure you serve warm or cold.

ASIAN CUCUMBER SESAME SALAD

PREP TIME25 minutes

INGREDIENTS

SALAD

2 large carrots

1 teaspoon of kosher salt

2 tablespoon of cilantro {chopped}

2 large seedless cucumbers

1 sweet pepper {chopped}

1 tablespoon of sesame seeds, white or black

1 green onion sliced, {**NOTE:** use the green part only for low FODMAP}

DRESSING

1 tablespoon of freshly squeezed lime juice, about ½ a lime

1 tablespoons of maple, can sub with honey or sugar

1 tablespoon of sesame oil

More salt to taste

2 tablespoon of rice vinegar

1 tablespoon of Coconut Aminos for paleo, or gluten free soy sauce/tamari

1 teaspoon of grated ginger

A pinch red pepper flakes, or to taste

Directions:

SALAD

1. First, trim the ends of the cucumber and spiralize the cucumbers or use a julienne peeler.
2. After which you place the sliced cucumbers in a colander and toss them with the 1 teaspoon of salt.
3. After that, let the cucumbers sit in the colander in the sink for at least 5 minutes to draw out excess water/moisture...
4. Then, while the cucumber is sitting, spiralize or peel the carrots and chop the sweet peppers. {NOTE: you can also use this time to prepare the dressing}.
5. Furthermore, once the cucumber has drained for 15 minutes, spread them out on a layer of paper towels, or a clean dish towel, and gently pat out as much moisture as you can.
6. At this point, place the cucumber noodles, carrots, and pepper in mixing bowl large enough to hold the salad.
7. This is when you add 2-3 tablespoons of the dressing and toss to combine, coating the salad.
8. Finally, top with sesame seeds, the sliced green onion, and cilantro and serve immediately.

NOTES

1. However, this salad is best eaten on the day of.
2. Remember, if you do save some for later make sure to store in an airtight container and you may need to drain some water before eating.

MCAULIFLOWER MASH

INGREDIENTS

1 onion {sliced}

A little sea salt and white pepper to season

1 cauliflower (approx 800g / 28 1/4 oz) finely chopped

1 clove garlic {smashed}

1 tablespoon of olive oil

Directions:

1. First, sauté onion and garlic in a large pot with the olive oil over a low to medium heat until softened.
2. After which you add the fine chopped cauliflower and ¼ cup water or vegetable stock.
3. After that, cover the pot completely with a tight fitting lid and turn down to heat to a low simmer.
4. Then, cook for about 5 - 10 minutes, stirring half way through and checking to make sure there is still enough liquid to steam the cauliflower. {NOTE: It's important not to overcook it to keep the fresh flavor intact}.
5. Furthermore, remove from the heat and place into a good high speed blender like a Vitamix.
6. This is when you season with a little sea salt and white pepper.
7. Finally, blend until smooth and creamy.
8. Make sure you serve hot and enjoy with your favorite comfort food dishes.

Pesto Zucchini Noodles with Asparagus

Ingredients for the pasta:

4 thick asparagus spears, with ends trimmed, sliced on an angle

¼ cup of jarred vegan pesto or better still homemade

1 teaspoon of extra virgin olive oil

Salt and pepper {to taste}

2 medium zucchinis, Blade D, noodles trimmed

Ingredients For the pesto:

1.5 tablespoons of pine nuts

Salt and pepper

1 large clove of garlic {minced}

3 cup of basil leaves {packed}

3-4 tablespoons of extra virgin olive oil

Directions:

1. Remember, if making homemade pesto, place all of the ingredients for the pesto into a food processor and pulse until creamy.
2. After which you taste and adjust, if necessary; set aside.
3. After that, heat the oil in a medium skillet over medium-high heat.
4. Then, once oil is shimmering, add in the asparagus and season generously with salt and pepper.
5. Furthermore, cook for about 5-7 minutes or until asparagus is bright green, fork tender, and is browned.

6. In the meantime, spiralize the zucchinis and place in a large mixing bowl.
7. After that, pour over the pesto and toss well; set aside.
8. At this point, when asparagus is done, toss it in the bowl with the pesto zucchini noodles and toss well to combine.
9. Finally, divide the pasta into bowls and serve.

Split Pea and Cauliflower Curry with Roasted Rutabaga Noodles

SERVES6

20 MINPREP TIME

40 MINCOOK TIME

Ingredients

½ red onion {peeled and diced}

2 carrots {peeled and diced}

1 large garlic clove {minced}

½ teaspoon of turmeric

½ teaspoon of ground coriander

1 teaspoon of ground ginger (or better still replace with 2 teaspoons fresh minced ginger)

1 head of cauliflower {chopped into small florets}

(2) 13.6oz cans lite coconut milk

3 small rutabagas or better still 2 large rutabagas

1 tablespoon of extra virgin olive oil

2 celery ribs {diced]

Salt and pepper {to taste}

1 ½ tablespoons of curry powder

1 teaspoon of cumin

1 teaspoon of chili powder

1 {28oz} can diced tomatoes {no salt added, drained}

1 cup of split peas

1 cup of vegetable broth

Directions:

1. Meanwhile, heat the oven to 425 degrees.
2. After which you heat the oil in a large pot over medium-high heat.
3. Then, once oil is shimmering, add the celery, onions, and carrots, season with salt and pepper, and cook for 3 minutes or until softened.
4. After that, add the garlic and stir until fragrant, about 30 seconds.
5. At this point, add the curry powder, cumin, turmeric, coriander and chili powder and stir until vegetables are coated in the spices.
6. Furthermore, add in the tomatoes, split peas, cauliflower, coconut milk, and broth and stir to combine well; season with salt. C
7. After which you cover and bring to a boil.
8. Then, once boiling, reduce heat to medium-low and let cook for 30-40 minutes or until peas are tender.
9. In addition, while curry cooks, line a baking sheet with parchment paper.
10. After that, peel and spiralize the rutabaga with Blade C. Lay out the rutabaga noodles, season with salt and pepper and bake in the oven for 10-15 minutes or until cooked through.
11. Finally, when curry is ready, divide the rutabaga noodles into bowls and top with curry.
12. Serve.

Avocado and Tomato Zucchini Noodle Salad with Basil Vinaigrette

20 MINPREP TIME

20 MINTOTAL TIME

Ingredients for the vinaigrette:

1 small garlic clove {peeled and chopped}

2 tablespoons of red wine vinegar

Salt {to taste}

1 pinch of red pepper flakes

1 ounce of fresh basil

¼ cup of olive oil

½ tablespoon of water

1 small shallot {chopped}

Ingredients for the salad:

1 cup of sun gold heirloom tomatoes (or better still cherry tomatoes), halved or sliced

Pepper {to taste}

2 medium zucchinis, Blade D, noodles trimmed

1 large ripe avocado {peeled, pitted and sliced into eight slivers}

1 cup of defrosted cooked green peas

Directions:

1. First, place the ingredients for the vinaigrette into a high speed blender and pulse until creamy, about 30 seconds; set aside.
2. After which you toss the zucchini noodles and tomatoes with three-quarters of the vinaigrette.
3. After that, divide the noodle mixture into four bowls and top each with two avocado slices and sprinkle over with peas.
4. Finally, pour over the remaining vinaigrette and season generously with pepper.

Roasted Fall Vegetable Salad with Kale and Brussels Slaw

Prep Time: 15

Cook Time: 30

Yield: 8

Tip:

This recipe is a hearty, healthy Roasted Fall Vegetable Salad with Maple Curry Vinaigrette on a bed of shredded kale and Brussels sprouts.

Ingredients

Roasted Fall Veggies

       3 small carrots {peeled}

       1 small yam

       Olive oil

       Generous pinch cumin seed and fennel seeds (it is optional)

       3 small parsnips {peeled}

       ½ a cauliflower

       1 small delicate squash

       Salt and pepper {to taste}

Salad

       8 ounces shredded Brussels sprouts (or slaw)

       1–2 cups of cooked lentils (little black caviar or French green)

1 bunch lacinato kale {stacked and thinly sliced}

1 tablespoon of olive oil

¼ teaspoon of salt

Optional additions –pumpkin seeds, golden raisins, (or better still maple glazed pecans), pomegranate seeds

Indian Curry Dressing

2 tablespoons of olive oil

2 tablespoons of maple syrup

1 teaspoon yellow curry powder; more to taste.

1 small shallot {finely diced}

3 tablespoons of apple cider vinegar

¼ teaspoon of salt

¼ teaspoon of pepper

Directions:

1. Meanwhile, heat oven to 425F
2. After which you cut parsnips and carrots into quarters, vertically, then half again if necessary, to get them to ½ inch thick at widest part.
3. After that, cut cauliflower into bit sized florets and yam (no need to peel) into ½ inch thick half-moons.
4. Then, split squash in half, remove seeds (no need to peel) and cut into ½ inch thick slices. (NOTE: Alternatively, you can cut them into rings, but will need to remove seeds from each ring.) P
5. Furthermore, place all the veggies on two, parchment lined sheet pans and drizzle with olive oil, sprinkle with salt and pepper. A

6. After which you add a pinch of the fennel and cumin seeds to the cauliflower; roast 30-35 minutes, tossing them halfway through.

7. At this point, place the shredded kale and Brussels sprouts in a large bowl and massage with olive oil and salt for about 3-4 minutes; add the lentils.

8. This is when you whisk the dressing ingredients together in a small bowl.

9. In addition, when veggies are done let them cool to room temp.

10. This is when you add them to the kale-Brussels sprout bowl and toss all with the curry dressing.

11. After which you taste, adjust salt and pepper. Remember, if you want a stronger curry flavor, I suggest you add more and toss it in.

12. Finally, top with seeds or nuts, golden raisins, and or pomegranate seeds.

13. Make sure you serve at room temp, or store in the fridge until ready to serve. NOTE: this salad keeps for several days.

Instant Pot Paleo Cauliflower Mushroom Risotto
(Whole30, Vegan, AIP)

Tip:

Remember, if you are looking for a quick and easy side dish, this Instant Pot Paleo Cauliflower Mushroom Risotto is so tasty and healthy and takes less than 30 minutes to prepare!

Prep Time5 mins

Cook Time14 mins

Pressurizing Time15 mins

Servings: 4 servings

Ingredients

1 tablespoon of ghee or coconut oil for AIP or dairy sensitivity

1 lb of small shiitake mushrooms, sliced or cremini or white mushrooms

2 tablespoons of coconut aminos

1 cup of bone broth or chicken broth or vegetable broth

1/2 teaspoon of sea salt or more, to taste

Chopped parsley {for garnish}

1 medium head of cauliflower or 4-5 cups of pre-riced fresh or frozen cauliflower

1 small onion {diced}

3 garlic cloves {minced}

1 cup of full-fat coconut milk

¼ cup of nutritional yeast

2 tablespoons of tapioca starch

Ground black pepper to taste (omit for AIP)

Directions:

1. First, remove the leaves off the cauliflower and cut off the florets from the roots.
2. After which you use a cheese grater or a food processor with a grater attachment, and grate the cauliflower into the size of rice.
3. After that, add ghee or coconut oil to the Instant Pot and set it to "Sauté." L
4. Then, let it heat for 5 minutes and make sure to coat the bottom of the pan.
5. Furthermore, add mushrooms, onion, and garlic and cook stirring for 7 minutes, until the mushrooms have sweat and are tender.
6. At this point, add coconut aminos, and stir cooking for 5 minutes until the vegetables are browned.
7. This is when you turn off the Instant Pot.
8. In addition, add coconut milk, cauliflower rice, bone broth, nutritional yeast, and sea salt; stir everything together.
9. After which you seal the lid, make sure the pressure valve is set to close, and set the Instant Pot to "Manual" for 2 minutes.
10. Then, once it finishes to a beep, immediately release the pressure valve and open the lid. However, you can drain some of the liquid if there's too much (NOTE: this depends on how much moisture was in your cauliflower).
11. Finally, sprinkle tapioca starch over the risotto and stir until thickened; add more salt if desired and ground black pepper, if using.
12. Make sure you serve warm, sprinkled with chopped parsley.

Spiral zed Butternut Squash with Creamy Cashew Alfredo

Serves 8

15 min Prep Time

15 min Cook Time

Ingredients

1/2 large onion {diced}

1 ¼ cups of unsweetened almond milk

¼ teaspoon of black pepper

2 large butternut squashes, spiral zed (it makes about 8 cups noodles)

2 cups of raw cashews

2 garlic cloves {minced}

3/4 teaspoon of salt

1 teaspoon of Dijon mustard

Juice of 1 lemon

Directions:

1. First, soak cashews overnight in 3 cups of water {NOTE: once soaked, drain completely}.
2. After which in a large pan over medium heat, sauté the onion and garlic until translucent.
3. At this point, remove from heat and allow cooling slightly.

4. Then, in a high-powered blender, blend soaked cashews, cooked onions and salt, pepper, garlic, almond milk, mustard, and lemon until very creamy; set aside.

5. In the meantime, sauté spiral zed squash in the same pan you used for the onions and garlic for about 10 minutes, or until cooked through.

6. Finally, pour in the Alfredo sauce, tossing to combine before serving!

Roasted Red Cabbage with Orange, Hazelnuts & Mint

Prep Time10 mins

Cook Time25 mins

Total Time35 mins

Servings: 6 slices

Ingredients

- 1 tablespoon of extra virgin olive oil

- 2 teaspoons of honey or maple syrup (omit if Whole30)

- 1 head red cabbage

- ¼ cup of chopped hazelnuts

- 2 tablespoons of orange juice

- 2 teaspoons of balsamic vinegar

- ¼ teaspoon of salt

- Zest from 1 orange

- 2 tablespoons of shredded fresh mint

Directions:

1. Meanwhile, heat the oven to 200 degrees Celsius (390 degrees Fahrenheit)
2. After which in a small sauce pan combine the olive oil, orange juice, balsamic and honey (or maple syrup) and bring to a boil on medium heat.
3. Then, once the mixture has boiled, reduce the heat to low.

4. At this point, cut the red cabbage into slices approximately 1/2 an inch thick, making sure that you include a portion of the stem in each slice so that the steaks hold together.

5. After that, lay the red cabbage slices on a baking sheet, sprinkle with salt and brush with some of the orange and balsamic liquid.

6. Furthermore, place in the oven and bake for approximately 20 to 25 minutes, removing from the oven and brushing with more liquid half way through cooking. {NOTE: the red cabbage is done when the stem of each slice is tender}.

7. Finally, place the red cabbage slices on a serving tray, brush with any remaining orange and balsamic liquid and top with the shredded mint, chopped hazelnuts and orange zest.

8. Enjoy!

Sweet Potato Pumpkin Fritters {Paleo, Whole30, Gluten Free, Vegan}

Makes about 16 small rounds

INGREDIENTS

¼ cup of pumpkin (I prefer this kind in the BPA-free carton)

¼ teaspoon of ground cinnamon

1/8 teaspoon of ground ginger

2 small sweet potatoes {about 2 cups}

3 tablespoons of coconut cream taken from the top of full-fat coconut milk

1/8 teaspoon of ground cardamom

¼ cup of coconut flour

1 tablespoon of coconut or better still avocado oil

Salt to taste

Directions:

1. First, steam sweet potatoes in Instant Pot; scrub the sweet potatoes, slice them lengthwise and then place them face down on the Instant Pot trivet. P
2. After which you pour 1 cup of water on the bottom, cover, hit steam for 3 minutes and let the air release naturally.
3. Let it cool and then scoop the flesh out into a bowl and discard the skin. NOTE: if you don't have an Instant Pot, I suggest you roast or steam your sweet potatoes on the stove until they're soft.
4. After that, place the steamed sweet potatoes, pumpkin, coconut cream and spices in a large glass bowl and mix until combined.
5. Then, gradually add the coconut flour to the mixture. Remember, it should be getting thick.

6.   Furthermore, form small patties with your hand. {NOTE: if the patties aren't staying together, you can add more flour}.
7.   After that, warm the coconut or avocado oil in a large skillet, over medium heat.
8.   Then, once warm, add the sweet potato pumpkin fritters and top with salt.

NOTE: don't crowd the pan; you want room to flip the fritters; work in batches.

9.   In addition, cook 5-10 minutes each side, or until golden brown.
10.   At this point, once both sides are crisp, remove from pan.
11.   Finally, top with my hemp lime cream or you can mix a little fresh lime juice with coconut yogurt.

Delectable Smoothie Recipes

Easy Pumpkin Pie Smoothie (Vegan, Dairy Free, Paleo-Friendly)

Ingredients

1 (about 13.5 ounce) can unsweetened coconut milk

1 banana, frozen (or better still regular banana with ½ cup ice)

1 Tablespoon of grass fed collagen powder (omit for vegan)

1 cup of pumpkin puree

1 teaspoon of pumpkin pie spice

3 Tablespoons of maple syrup, to taste (or better still raw honey, or other sweetener, optional) *

Directions:

1. First, add coconut milk to blender, and then add remaining ingredients.
2. After which you blend on HIGH for 1 minute, or until smooth.
3. Then, serve with a sprinkle of cinnamon or whipped cream, if desired.

Notes

You can sub alternate sweeteners including stevia, raw honey, erythritol, etc.

MIXED BERRY SMOOTHIE RECIPE (WHOLE30, PALEO, VEGAN)

Ingredients

1/2-3/4 cup of milk of choice

1 frozen banana {optional}

1 cup of frozen mixed berries

1 tablespoon of chia seeds

1-2 tablespoons of cashew butter can substitute for any nut or seed butter of choice

Directions:

First, add all ingredients into the blender and blend until desired consistency. NOTE: for a thicker, ice cream like smoothie, I suggest you blend less. Remember, if smoothie is too thick, add more milk of choice.

Notes

1.   For thinner smoothies, I suggest you add more milk as needed
2.   This smoothie can be chilled for 30 minutes or so.

PALEO GREEN SMOOTHIE

This recipe is packed with fiber and naturally sweetened with fresh fruit. Simply blend and enjoy the healthiest green smoothie ever!

Serving: Makes about 600 ml (2 ½ cups)

INGREDIENTS

2 cups of curly kale

1 medium banana {fresh or frozen}

1 tablespoon of chia seeds

1 to 1 ¼ cups of ice

½ to 1 cup of dairy-free milk from a carton

4 cups of baby spinach

6 pieces' strawberries, {fresh or frozen}

2 teaspoons of hemp seeds {it is optional}

Directions:

1. First, place everything in a high speed blender in the order listed in the recipe.
2. After which you blend 1 minute or until creamy smooth. A
3. Then, add more milk or ice cubes for thinner smoothie.

STRAWBERRY BANANA SMOOTHIE BOWL

Tip:

This recipe is a simple and sweet treat! It's a healthy Paleo + vegan breakfast or snack made with only a few ingredients and feel free to add whichever toppings your heart desires to customize to your tastes.

INGREDIENTS

Ingredients for the smoothie bowl

1½ cups of frozen strawberries

½ cup of Silk Unsweetened Coconut Milk

1 banana {frozen}

Ingredients for the toppings

Fresh strawberries {sliced}

Chia seeds

Simple Truth Freeze Dried Strawberries + Bananas

Fresh bananas {sliced}

Directions:

1. First, combine frozen strawberries, frozen banana, and coconut milk in a blender (I prefer my Vitamix).
2. After which you puree until completely smooth – the mixture should be thick. A
3. After that, add a touch more liquid if necessary to get it to blend completely smooth.
4. Then, transfer to a bowl and add toppings as desired.
5. Enjoy!

Healthy Mixed Berry Smoothie (Whole30, Paleo, Vegan)

Tips:

This recipe is a thick, creamy and filling mixed berry breakfast smoothie using just four ingredients and naturally sweetened! Easy, quick and extremely satisfying, this recipe is packed with fiber, protein, and fruit, and is naturally vegan, paleo, gluten free, dairy free and whole30 friendly!

Prep Time1 minute

Cook Time2 minutes

Servings1 smoothie

Ingredients

1/2-3/4 cup of milk of choice

1 frozen banana {it is optional}

1 cup of frozen mixed berries

1-2 tablespoons of cashew butter can substitute for any nut or seed butter of choice

1 tablespoon of chia seeds

Directions:

First, add all ingredients into the blender and blend until desired consistency.

NOTE:

1.   For a thicker, ice cream like smoothie, I suggest you blend less.
2.   However, if smoothie is too thick, add more milk of choice.
3.   Add more milk as needed, For thinner smoothies

4. This smoothie can be chilled for 30 minutes or so, for an even thicker smoothie.

Paleo blueberry banana chia

Yield: 2 smoothies (about 4 cups)

Tip:

This is a 4-ingredient recipe for antioxidant-rich and refreshing blueberry banana chia smoothies.

INGREDIENTS

1 ½ cups unsweetened almond milk {divided}

1 ½ cups of frozen blueberries

2 tablespoons of chia seeds

3 medium bananas {sliced and frozen}

Directions:

1. First, in a small bowl, add chia seeds and ½ cup almond milk.
2. After which you whisk until thoroughly combined.
3. After that, cover and chill in the refrigerator for about 10 minutes.
4. Then, add bananas and remaining 1 cup almond milk to a blender.
5. At this point, blend until smooth, scraping down the sides of the blender as needed.
6. This is when you add blueberries, blending until smooth.
7. Furthermore, remove the chia seed mixture from the refrigerator—it should have thickened to a gel-like consistency.
8. After that, whisk until well mixed.
9. Then, using a rubber spatula or spoon, scrape the chia seed mixture into the blender.
10. Make sure you blend until smooth.
11. Finally, pour into two cups.
12. Enjoy immediately!

Easy berry smoothie recipe

Prep Time: 5 mins

Cook Time: 0 mins

Yield: 2 smoothies

Tips:

This recipe is quick & easy berry smoothie is ready in 5 minutes!

It is refreshing, packed with antioxidants and delicious.

INGREDIENTS

Easy Berry Smoothie

> 1 cup of unsweetened almond milk
>
> 1 cup of frozen blueberries
>
> 1–2 scoops vegan vanilla protein powder (it is optional)
>
> 2 medium bananas {sliced and frozen}
>
> 1 cup of frozen strawberries
>
> 1 cup of frozen raspberries

Directions:

1. First, add bananas into a blender or food processor.
2. After which you blend until the bananas become crumbly; add almond milk.
3. After that, blend until smooth and creamy, scraping down the sides of the blender as needed.
4. Then, add blueberries, strawberries, and raspberries. B

5. Furthermore, blend until smooth, again scraping down the sides of the blender as needed.
6. Finally, pour into two cups and enjoy!

Strawberry banana smoothie bowl (paleo + vegan)

Prep Time: 5 minutes

Yield: 1 bowl

Tips:

1. This recipe is a simple and sweet treat!
2. It's a healthy Paleo + vegan breakfast or snack made with but a few ingredients, and feel free to add whichever toppings your heart desires to customize to your tastes.

INGREDIENTS

FOR THE SMOOTHIE BOWL

1½ cups of frozen strawberries

½ cup of Silk Unsweetened Coconut Milk

1 banana {frozen}

FOR THE TOPPINGS

Fresh strawberries {sliced}

Simple Truth Freeze Dried Strawberries + Bananas

Chia seeds

Fresh bananas {sliced}

Directions:

1. First, combine frozen strawberries, frozen banana, and coconut milk in a blender (I prefer my Vitamix).
2. After which you puree until completely smooth – the mixture should be thick.

3. Then, add a touch more liquid if necessary to get it to blend completely smooth.
4. Finally, transfer to a bowl and add toppings as desired.
5. Enjoy!

Banana date smoothie bowl

Prep Time: 5 minutes

Yield: 1 bowl 1x

Tips:

1. This recipe is a creamy and sweet treat that tastes like ice cream but is simple and healthy enough for breakfast thanks to a secret veggie that's snuck in there.
2. However, it is time to make you a bowl of this paleo and vegan banana date goodness on the next warm morning for a refreshing breakfast.

INGREDIENTS

1 banana {frozen}

1 Medjool date {pitted}

1 tablespoon of flax seeds

½ cup of almond milk

½ cup of frozen cauliflower {NOTE: steam before freezing for the best flavor}

1 tablespoon of almond butter

Optional: ½ teaspoon vanilla extract and/or better still ½ teaspoon cinnamon

Directions:

1. First, combine all of the ingredients in a blender (I prefer my Vitamix).
2. After which you blend until smooth + garnish with freeze-dried bananas, almond butter, flax seeds, berries of choice, and/or whatever other goodness you feel like!

Kid-Friendly Smoothie Bowls (Vegan, Paleo)

PREP TIME5 MINUTES

SERVINGS2

Ingredients

Dragon Fruit Bowl:

> 1 large banana
>
> 1/2 cup of frozen raspberries or strawberries
>
> 2 tablespoons of apple juice optional
>
> 1 frozen packet of pitaya
>
> 1/3 cup of unsweetened almond or nut milk
>
> 1 tablespoon of chia seeds

Acai Bowl:

> 1 large banana
>
> 1 tablespoon of almond butter
>
> 2-3 tablespoons of apple juice optional
>
> 1 frozen packet of acai
>
> ½ cup of frozen strawberries or blueberries
>
> 1/2 unsweetened almond milk or better still nut milk
>
> 1 tablespoon of hemp seeds

Additional toppings:

1/2 cup of fresh strawberries

1/4 cup of flaked or better still shredded coconut

1 kiwi {sliced}

1/3 cup of fresh blueberries

Directions:

1. First, choose between the dragon fruit or acai smoothie bowl, and place those ingredients into a high powered blender.
2. After which you pulse until smooth.
3. Then, adjust for sweetness by adding in apple juice.
4. Finally, top with fresh fruit, nuts, coconut, seeds, bananas, or even granola.

Sweet Potato Smoothie (Paleo/Vegan)

Prep Time5 minutes

Servings1

Ingredients

1 cup of frozen cauliflower rice (about 100 grams)

½ teaspoon of vanilla extract

¼ teaspoon of nutmeg

1 ½ cups of unsweetened vanilla almond milk (or more or less depending on smoothie thickness preference)

1 small sweet potato baked, cut, and frozen* (about 6.5 ounces/1 ½ cups cubed)

1 tablespoon of almond butter

1/2 tablespoon of cinnamon

1 teaspoon of maple syrup (optional)

Optional additions: collagen, chia seeds, protein powder, yogurt...

Directions:

1.   First, put all ingredients to a Vitamix or high powdered blender and blend until smooth, about 1 minute.
2.   Then, top with toppings or drink as it.

Notes

1. Remember, for you to bake sweet potato, preheat oven to 400 degrees and bake from 30-40 minutes until soft and can be pierced with a knife.
2. Then, cut into large cubes and place in the freezer until frozen solid.

Vanilla Cheesecake Paleo Smoothie with Protein {Vegan, No Added Sugar}

Tip:

1. This amazingly delicious recipe is loaded with good stuff and it's sweetened with dates and is completely paleo, dairy free, and vegan.
2. You can add a scoop of your favorite protein or collagen for a nourishing snack or dessert!

Prep Time: 5 minutes

Servings: 4

Ingredients

4 medjool dates pitted (**NOTE:** softened first, if necessary)

½ cup unsweetened almond milk

2 1/2 Tablespoons of fresh lemon juice about 1 lemon

Crumbled vanilla wafer cookies {it is optional}

2/3 cup of raw cashews {**NOTE:** I did not soak them first but you can if you prefer}

3/4 cup of full fat coconut milk

2 teaspoons of pure vanilla extract

Handful ice

1 scoop of protein powder or collagen peptides optimal

Directions:

1. First, place all ingredients (except for the cookie crumbles) in a high speed blender and blend until very smooth.
2. Then, serve right away topped with cookie crumbles if desired

Notes

1. Remember, if you use all coconut milk; make sure it's the "light" version since full fat will be too thick.
2. However, using all almond milk will result in a thinner, less creamy smoothie.
3. For vegan cookie crumbles, I suggest you use my n'oatmeal raisin cookie recipe without the raisins!

CLASSIC GREEN SMARTER SMOOTHIE {KETO, PALEO, VEGAN-OPTION}

Serves: it is one very large serving or two smaller servings

Ingredients

1 very large handful spinach

¼ cup of blueberries (feel free to add a little more if this is serving two)

½ avocado

Sprinkle shredded coconut on top

2 cups of unsweetened almond milk (or better still other non-dairy milk)

1 very large handful frozen zucchini (NOTE: it can also be fresh)

1-2 heaping scoops of vanilla protein (NOTE: two scoops for two servings)

1 tablespoon of chia seeds

Directions:

1. First, starting with the liquid first, add all of the ingredients to your high speed blender.
2. After which you blend until smooth and creamy.
3. Then, serve topped with your coconut or other crunchies on top!

Cookie Dough Smoothie (Paleo, Vegan)

Prep Time: 10 minutes

Cook Time: 0 minutes

Yield: serves 1-2 1x

Tip:

This recipe tastes like ice cream, but is healthy, nourishing, and high in protein and contains hidden veggies and it's perfect for any meal of the day!

Ingredients

½ heaping cup frozen cubed sweet potato (about 80g)

2 scoops of vanilla protein powder

Handful chocolate chips

1 heaping cup frozen cauliflower florets (about 125g)

½ ripe banana (about 75g)

1 heaping Tablespoons of almond butter (preferably sunflower seed butter for nut free)

Plant based milk (add 1 Tablespoon at a time, as needed)

Directions:

1. First, slightly defrost frozen cauliflower and sweet potato by warming in the microwave for 15 seconds.
2. After that, in a food processor or high powered blender, blend cauliflower, sweet potato and banana for a few seconds.
3. After which you stop to scrape the sides, and then blend a few seconds more.

4. Furthermore, add in remaining ingredients (except chocolate chips) and blend until smooth, stopping to scrape the sides every so often.

5. At this point, add more liquid as needed.

6. This is when you add chocolate chips to the smoothie and pulse a few times until combined.

7. Finally, scoop smoothie into a bowl and eat!

Green Protein Smoothie (Vegan + Paleo)

Yield: 2

Prep time: 6 MINUTES

Tip:

This is one of the healthiest, yet most delicious, green smoothies I've tried!

Ingredients

1 cup of spinach

1 thumb-sized piece of fresh ginger {peeled}

1 heaped tablespoon of hemp protein

1 1/2 cups of unsweetened almond milk

2 cups of chopped mango

2 small green apples, chopped (skins on, core removed)

2 tablespoons of chia seeds

1 teaspoon of spirulina powder

Directions:

1. First, add everything to a high-powered blender and mix until smooth. A
2. After which you add some ice cubes if you want to help make it colder and thicker.
3. Then, taste and adjust, if needed. NOTE: if it's too thick, I suggest you add more almond milk.
4. Finally, pour into two large glasses.
5. Serve and enjoy!

Notes

However, if you're unsure of the taste of spirulina, as it can be quite strong, start with 1/2 teaspoon and work your way up. Feel free to add up to a tablespoon!

No grains or refined Green Smoothie Bowl: Paleo, Vegan

Tips:

This Delicious recipe is great to start a day with its goodness of spinach, banana, green grapes, and mango, avocado and almond milk.

Prep Time5 mins

Servings: 1

Ingredients

1 banana

¼ cup of unsweetened almond milk

½ cup of green grapes

1 ½ cup of spinach {packed}

½ cup of chopped mango {or small mango}

½ avocado

Topping

Blueberries

Hempseeds

Banana

Mango

Directions:

1. First, in a blender or food processor process all ingredients for smoothie bowl into fine consistency and transfer to a bowl and top with toppings.

2. Enjoy.

Awakening Matcha Smoothie Bowl Recipe

Tip:

This refreshing recipe fuses super foods match a, chia and pomegranate for a satisfying and healthy, how to best kick start your day.

Ingredients

2 cups of unsweetened almond milk

1/2 cup of unsweetened coconut flakes

1 Tablespoon of chia seeds

3 large frozen bananas {sliced into chunks}

2 Tablespoons of match a green tea powder

1/2 cup of raspberries

1/2 cup of pomegranate arils

Directions:

1. First, place almond milk, frozen banana, and match a powder in a blender.
2. After which you blend on high until smooth.
3. Then, divide smoothie between two bowls.
4. Finally, top each bowl with pomegranate arils, raspberries, chia seeds and coconut flakes or toppings of your choice.
5. Enjoy right away.

Pineapple Green Smoothie

Prep Time: 5 minutes

Cook Time: 0 minutes

Yield: 1 smoothie 1x

Tips:

This recipe is made with only 5 ingredients! I

However, it's packed with minerals, vitamins, antioxidants and will help keep you full and hydrated between meals.

Ingredients

1 cup of baby spinach leaves

1 Tablespoon of hemp hearts

1 cup of unsweetened full fat coconut milk

1 cup of frozen pineapple (feel free to use fresh in the same quantity but won't end up with a cold smoothie)

1 pitted medjool date

Directions:

1. First, blend all ingredients in a high speed blender until smooth.
2. Then pour, drink and enjoy!

CINNAMON PEANUT BUTTER SMOOTHIE

INGREDIENTS

1/3 cup of almond butter, or better still organic peanut butter, if you want

1 cup of milk of choice (I prefer to use my homemade coconut milk)

2 cups of ice

2-3 ripe bananas

1/2 cup of applesauce (it is optional)

1 tablespoon of chia seeds

1 teaspoon of cinnamon

Directions:

First, combine all ingredients in blender and blend on high until smooth

Chocolate Avocado Smoothie

Tips:

This recipe tastes like a rich chocolate milkshake, while being dairy-free and naturally sweetened with fruit.

PREP TIME5 minutes

SERVINGS1

INGREDIENTS

> 4 Medjool dates {pitted}
>
> 1 heaping tablespoons of cacao powder
>
> 1 heaping cup of ice cubes
>
> 3/4 cup of water
>
> ¼ avocado
>
> ½ teaspoon of vanilla extract
>
> 1 handful fresh baby spinach (it is optional)

Directions:

1. First, in a high-speed blender, combine the dates, water, cacao powder, avocado, vanilla, and spinach, if using, and blend until very smooth.
2. After which you taste the pudding-like mixture to make sure there's enough sweetness and chocolate flavor to your liking, and adjust anything to your taste. (**NOTE:** Keep in mind that the flavor will be diluted a bit more once you add the ice.)

3. After that, add the ice and blend again, until the smoothie has more of a milkshake-like texture. Remember, you can add as much ice as needed to achieve the texture you want, but keep in mind that extra ice will dilute the chocolate flavor.

4. Then, serve right away.

Whole30 Cherry Smoothie

Tips:

This protein powder and banana-free makes a healthy snack or delicious treat.

Prep Time 5 minutes

Cook Time 0 minutes

Servings 2 small

Ingredients

>3 ice cubes
>
>1 tablespoon of Chia Seeds
>
>1 tablespoon of cashew butter
>
>1/4 teaspoon of chlorella powder optional
>
>½ cup of water
>
>3/4 cup of frozen cherries
>
>2 tablespoons of cacao powder
>
>2 tablespoon of maple syrup
>
>2 dates
>
>½ cup of almond milk

Directions:

1. First, in a powerful blender add the cherries and ice cubes.
2. After which you pulse slightly to chop.

3.   After that, add in the remaining ingredients.
4.   Then, pour the almond milk and water on top.
5.   Finally, blend until smooth.

Paleo Key Lime Pie Smoothie

Prep Time 5 minutes

Servings 2

Ingredients

¼ cup of macadamia nuts OR better still raw cashews (more carbs), soaked if you do not have a high power blender to pulverize

1/2 medium avocado

1 tablespoon of erythritol or any favorite low carb sweetener to taste, or better still honey, or a banana (last 2 NOT keto)

2 tablespoons of collagen {this is the brand I use, use tessa10 for 10% any order}

Zest of one lime

2 cups of coconut milk {I prefer Trader Joe's Coconut Milk, unsweetened. Feel free to add some of my favorite canned milk variety for extra healthy fats too!}

4 tablespoons of lime juice

Two handfuls of spinach or any greens. {NOTE: I also sometimes add a handful of raw cauliflower}.

2 tablespoons of coconut butter I use my homemade,

Splash vanilla extract optional

Directions:

First, place all ingredients into a blender and whir until smooth and creamy.

Orange Carrot Smoothie with Ginger

SERVES: 1

PREP:5 minutes

INGREDIENTS

> 3/4 Cup of Orange juice
>
> Honey (it is Optional and to taste)
>
> 1 Cup of Ice cubes
>
> 1/3 Cup of Carrot {sliced}
>
> 1 teaspoon of Fresh ginger {minced}

Direction:

First, place all ingredients into a high-powered blender and blend until smooth!

Paleo and Vegan 5 Ingredient Pineapple Banana Smoothie

Prep time 5 mins

Serves: 2½ cups

Ingredients

1 large banana {peeled and sliced}

1 – 2 tablespoons of pure maple syrup (feel free to sub raw honey, but honey isn't vegan)

¼ - ½ teaspoon of organic ground ginger (it is optional) (you can also use cinnamon, preferably Ceylon cinnamon)

1 cup of fresh pineapple chunks

1 ½ cups of unsweetened vanilla almond milk (feel free to sub another non-diary milk of choice)

¼ teaspoon of pure vanilla extract

Directions:

1. First, in a large high-speed food processor or blender, add all the ingredients.
2. After that, blend until it's smooth and creamy.
3. Then, serve and enjoy!

Purple Power Smoothie Bowls (Paleo)

Prep Time: 15 minutes

Total Time: 15 minutes

Servings: 2 servings

Ingredients

1 cup of frozen blueberries

½ cup of blackberries

½ medium banana fresh or frozen

2 ounces' protein powder of choice, vanilla or better still chocolate optional

1 cup of beets, peeled and diced

1 cup of frozen raspberries plus more for topping

1 cup of carton coconut milk

1/2 medium avocado {skin and pit removed}

1 Tablespoon of pure maple syrup

Toppings:

Coconut milk

Unsweetened shredded coconut

Rolled oats or granola

Additional raspberries, blueberries, or blackberries

Directions:

1.   First, in a blender, combine all the ingredients and blend until smooth.

NOTE: for an extra thick smoothie bowl and for additional protein, I suggest you add a scoop of protein powder to this smoothie bowl if you like.

2.   After that, add the protein powder and blend again.
3.   Then, pour into 2 bowls and top with your choice of toppings.
4.   Make sure you serve immediately.
5.   Enjoy!

Notes

1.   Feel free to use either cooked beets or raw beets.
2.   Remember, for a creamier smoothie bowl, use cooked beets

Chocolate Avocado Smoothie (paleo, vegan, dairy-free options)

Prep Time: 3 min

Cook Time: 0 min

Yield: 1 large smoothie

Ingredients

2 tablespoons of Dutch-process cocoa powder

¼ cup of plain Greek yogurt or coconut cream for the paleo / vegan option

1/2 teaspoon of vanilla extract

85 grams' cold avocado flesh (about ~ 1/2 Hass avocado)

1 medium cold banana (NOTE: mine was 120 grams without the peel)

2-4 tablespoons of milk, optional (NOTE: for vegan, dairy-free, or paleo - use non-dairy milk)

Directions

1. First, blend everything together in a food processor (or better still a blender if you have a very good one - mine requires too much liquid for a thick smoothie like this) until it's very creamy.
2. After which you add more milk until it's the desired thickness.
3. Then, serve immediately or keep covered in the refrigerator for up to one day.

Notes

However, coconut cream (from a can of refrigerated canned coconut milk) or better still coconut milk yogurt will yield a thick smoothie but you could also use coconut milk for a thinner version.

Creamy pink smoothie bowl (vegan + paleo + refined sugar-free)

Prep Time: 7

Total Time: 7

Yield: 1-2 1x

Tips:

1. However, this vegan smoothie bowl is sweet, tart and super thick. I
2. Remember, that it has fun toppings that complement the flavors of the nutritious smoothie base; the base is mainly raspberries and bananas.
3. In addition, the raspberries offer dietary fiber, vitamin C and the bananas are a good source of vitamin C, vitamin B6 and fiber.

INGREDIENTS

1 teaspoon of vanilla extract

2 frozen sliced bananas

1/2 cup of unsweetened, plain plant-based milk (I recommend almond milk)

4 large pitted Medjool dates (or better still substitute 2 tablespoons pure maple syrup)

1/4 cup of blanched and slivered almonds or raw cashews

1 cup of frozen raspberries

Boost it with: 1 tablespoon of chia seeds, hemp seeds and/or ground flaxseed

Toppings:

Raw chunky almond butter (I prefer Trader Joe's brand)

Unsweetened shredded coconut

Raspberry chia jam

Dragon fruit (pitaya), thinly sliced and cut into stars with vegetable cutters

Frozen berries

Directions:

1. First, in a high speed blender, add all the ingredients except the frozen raspberries.
2. After which you blend until smooth and creamy.
3. After that, add the frozen raspberries and blend again until no chunks remain.
4. Then, taste and adjust sweetness and flavors as desired. P
5. Finally, pour into 1-2 shallow bowls and garnish as shown in the picture. Or, be creative and do your own thing.

NOTES

Note: however, if you need to use more milk to get the blender going try adding only a little bit at a time and if you use too much the smoothie bowl will lose its creaminess and thickness.

Paleo Caribbean Sunset Smoothie

Tips:

This recipe will make you feel like you're in the tropics.

It is a light, delicious and nutritious all natural drink!

Serves: 24 ounces

Ingredients

> 1 cup of frozen strawberries
>
> 1 ½ cups of orange juice {preferably freshly squeezed}
>
> 1 frozen banana
>
> 1 cup of ripe papaya

Directions:

First, place all ingredients in blender and blend on high until smooth.

Notes: things you will need

> **Measuring cups**
>
> **High-speed blender**

Dairy-Free Raspberry Smoothie Bowls

Prep time 5 mins

Total time 5 mins

Serves: 2 servings

Ingredients

2 cups of frozen raspberries

1 tablespoon of chia seeds

Raspberry Smoothie Bowl

1 large frozen banana

⅔ Cup of lite canned coconut milk, plus additional if needed

Optional Toppings

Shredded coconut

Chopped hazelnuts

Edible flowers

Fresh raspberries

Shaved dark chocolate

Chia seeds

Directions:

1. First, in a blender, puree the banana, raspberries, coconut milk, and chia seeds until smooth. NOTE: the mixture will be very thick. S
2. This is when you stop and push down the ingredients, as needed, and if necessary, add more coconut milk.

3. Then, scrape the smoothie into two bowls, and garnish with any or all of the optional toppings, as desired.

VEGAN CHOCOLATE RASPBERRY SMOOTHIE

PREP TIME5 minutes

TOTAL TIME5 minutes

INGREDIENTS

1 cup of fresh papaya and raspberry

1 tablespoon of cacao powder

1 cup of Cauliflower (Steamed then Frozen)

1 tablespoon of chia seeds

1/2 cup of nut milk

Directions:

1. First, blend everything together
2. Then, add toppings of your choice: I like coconut flakes, granola, cacao nibs, berries

NOTES

However, if you soak chia seeds in the nut milk first for 5-10 min (it turns into chia pudding), then you blend everything else in, the smoothie will turn out creamier.

Pumpkin Pie Smoothie (Paleo, Vegan, Dairy-Free)

PREP TIME5 minutes

Ingredients

1 (about 13.5 ounce) can unsweetened coconut milk

1 banana, frozen (or better still regular banana with ½ cup ice)

1 Tablespoon grass fed collagen powder (omit for vegan)

1 cup of pumpkin puree

1 teaspoon of pumpkin pie spice

3 Tablespoons of maple syrup, to taste (or better still raw honey, or other sweetener, it is optional) *

Directions:

First, add coconut milk to blender, after which you add remaining ingredients.

After that, blend on HIGH for 1 minute, or until smooth.

Then, serve with a sprinkle of cinnamon or whipped cream, if desired.

Notes

You can sub alternate sweeteners including stevia, raw honey, erythritol, etc.

Banana & almond breakfast shake {3-ingredients, paleo, vegan}

INGREDIENTS

8 whole almonds

1–1/2 medium-large, ripe bananas {frozen}

2/3 cup of nondairy milk (I prefer almond milk)

Optional: large pinch of ground cinnamon

Directions:

1. First, cut the frozen banana into pieces. A
2. After which you add all of the ingredients to a blender and blend until thick and smooth.
3. Serve immediately.

PINEAPPLE MANGO SMOOTHIE

Prep Time: 10 mins

Cook Time: 5 mins

Yield: 2 servings 1x

INGREDIENTS

1/2 cup of almond milk (or better still other milk of your choosing)

1 cup of frozen pineapple chunks

3 tablespoons of agave nectar (vegan) or better still 100% pure honey (paleo), optional

1/2 cup of ice cubes

1 mango {peeled and sliced}

3 mandarin oranges {peeled}

Directions:

1. First, add ingredients to blender in the order listed.
2. After which you blend on medium to high speed until smooth.
3. Then, top with fresh fruit, chia seeds, or leave as is.

Vegan Detox Green Monster Smoothie

PREP TIME5 MINUTES

TOTAL TIME5 MINUTES

SERVES1

Ingredients

1/2 cup of cucumber {peeled and sliced}

1 cup of vanilla almond milk (or alternate milk)

Large handful of spinach

¾ cup of frozen strawberries.

1 large frozen banana {broken into pieces}

1 ½ cups kale, loosely packed, stems removed (you can also use spinach)

Directions:

1. First, add the almond milk to a high-power blender and toss the banana pieces and kale in; blend on high.
2. After which you add the strawberries and cucumber.
3. After that, blend again until smooth.
4. Then, add in more almond milk and/or ice for desired consistency.

www.ingramcontent.com/pod-product-compliance
Lightning Source LLC
Chambersburg PA
BHW080420030426
335CB00020B/2523